Ultra Wideband Wireless Body Area Networks

Kasun Maduranga Silva Thotahewa
Jean-Michel Redouté · Mehmet Rasit Yuce

Ultra Wideband Wireless Body Area Networks

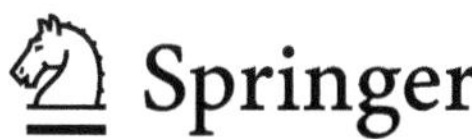 Springer

Kasun Maduranga Silva Thotahewa
Jean-Michel Redouté
Mehmet Rasit Yuce
Electrical and Computer Systems
    Engineering
Monash University
Melbourne, VIC
Australia

ISBN 978-3-319-35300-5   ISBN 978-3-319-05287-8   (eBook)
DOI 10.1007/978-3-319-05287-8
Springer Cham Heidelberg New York Dordrecht London

Printed on acid-free paper

Springer is part of Springer Science+Business Media (www.springer.com)

Preface

Wireless Body Area Network (WBAN) is an emerging networking concept that facilitates data communication using wearable and implantable sensor nodes. Wireless health monitoring is a key area of use for WBAN technology. WBAN communication systems can be easily incorporated into health care and home environments providing various advantages, such as avoiding the requirement to visit healthcare facilities for health monitoring, providing patients with an opportunity to keep a personal health record, and possibility of monitoring health information when the patient is involved in daily activities. Wearable and implantable communication devices involved in a WBAN require having small form factor, low power consumption, and scalable data rates ranging from Kbps to Mbps. Low cost, simple hardware implementation, and low processing power are also key requirements for sensor nodes in a WBAN. Impulse Radio-Ultra-Wideband (IR-UWB) can be considered as an attractive wireless technology for WBAN applications due to its inherent features, such as low power consuming transmitter design, low complexity hardware implementation, possibility of developing sensor nodes with small form factors, and high data rate capability.

This book discusses the current state of the art in the IR-UWB technology for WBAN applications. The book systematically introduces some of the existing IR-UWB-based WBAN design techniques. It provides a comprehensive review of the current MAC protocol designs for UWB-based WBAN applications. It also presents a detailed discussion on various hardware designs used in UWB transceiver design. An IR-UWB-based communication system has to be designed in a manner such that it enhances the advantages provided by IR-UWB transmitters while avoiding the complexities introduced by IR-UWB receivers. This book presents a comprehensive description on implementation of a dual-band communication system that uses IR-UWB for data transmission from sensor nodes while using narrowband technology for data reception.

The initial chapters of the book describe the design and evaluation of a dual-band MAC protocol for WBAN sensor nodes. A simulation-based performance analysis of this MAC protocol is presented in terms of critical parameters, such as packet error rate, throughput, packet delay, and power consumption. The latter half of the book describes the implementation and evaluation of a complete communication platform for WBAN applications that includes sensor nodes, coordinator nodes, and interfacing computer software. Wireless communication for implantable devices is another potential area for the use of the IR-UWB technology in WBAN applications. The last chapter of the book is dedicated to describe a feasibility study on the suitability of IR-UWB technology for implant applications. This study is focused on electromagnetic and thermal power absorption of human tissue that is exposed to IR-UWB signals. The outcomes of this study can be used as a guide in designing IR-UWB systems for implant applications.

We believe that this book will assist students and researchers who work in the area of UWB-based wireless communication. Especially, the hardware design of the UWB system in this book is presented in a manner such that the readers will be able to reproduce the hardware following the information given in the book. We firmly believe that it will assist in developing experimental UWB systems using off-the-shelf components for research purposes. Finally, we would like to thank all the parties who assisted us in producing this book. Our especial gratitude extends to Dr. Tharaka Dissanayake for his assistance with the UWB antennas. We are grateful to the Department of Electrical and Computer Systems Engineering, Monash University, Australia for providing us with the research facilities. We would also like to thank the publisher for providing us with the opportunity of delivering this book to a broad audience.

Kasun Maduranga Silva Thotahewa
Jean-Michel Redouté
Mehmet Rasit Yuce

Contents

Chapter 1
Wireless Body Area Network and Ultra-Wideband Communication

Abstract Current healthcare systems face new challenges due to the ageing population in the world. Aged population (over 65 years) has become a significant proportion of the total population in most of the countries. According to the World Health Organization (WHO), one in every four people will be over 65 years by 2056 [1]. With increasing demand for healthcare facilities, researchers have paid their attention towards improving existing healthcare infrastructure. Mobile healthcare has become a lucrative area in the eyes of researchers as well as entrepreneurs. Non-invasive and ambulatory health monitoring has become increasingly popular in modern healthcare as a solution for the increasing demand for hospital facilities. It has gained popularity not only for patient monitoring, but also in the field of sports where vital signs of sportsmen are monitored while they are on the field [2]. Ability to remotely monitor patients has many benefits. It is a solution for the increasing demand for physical infrastructure at hospitals. With the use of mobile health facilities, the requirement of patients being physically present in a hospital is eliminated. Vital body information can be transferred to a remote database via internet. Since the patients are monitored in real time while they are involved in their day to day activities, obtained parameters give more realistic overview of patient's health status. Consider a patient with high blood pressure; if it is possible to remotely monitor his/her blood pressure throughout the day, physicians can get a more realistic idea how the blood pressure builds up prior to reaching a certain threshold. Also it can eliminate inaccurate results caused by changed physical conditions that occur due to travelling to a hospital. It also makes it easy to keep track of the patient's or sportsman's health history. An early health warning system can also be implemented using this technology. An efficient Wireless Body Area Network (WBAN) is able to provide all the aforementioned benefits to both patients and physicians.

Keywords IR-UWB · WBAN · Transceivers · Patient monitoring · WPAN · WLAN · Zigbee · Bluetooth · UWB advantages

K. M. S. Thotahewa et al., *Ultra Wideband Wireless Body Area Networks*,
DOI: 10.1007/978-3-319-05287-8_1,
© Springer International Publishing Switzerland 2014

1.1 Overview of Wireless Body Area Networks

With the recent advancement in wireless sensor networks and miniaturized hardware technologies, it has been possible to implement wireless networks that operate in and around human body. A WBAN is a networking concept that has evolved with the idea of monitoring vital physiological signals from low power and miniaturized in-body or on-body sensors. Data collected from these sensors are transferred to a remote node via a wireless medium, where the data is forwarded to a higher layer application to be interpreted.

WBAN communication can be divided into three major categories; communication between a node on body surface to an outside base station, communication between two nodes that are placed on body surface, and communication from a node that is implanted in the body to an outside node. These three communication scenarios are named off-body communication, on-body communication and in-body communication respectively [3]. The IEEE wireless body area network standard (IEEE 804.15.6 TG6) [4] had been formed in order to develop and standardize the Physical Layer (PHY) and Medium Access Control (MAC) protocols for short range, low power and highly reliable wireless communication schemes to operate in, on and around the human body. The recent activities of this standard can be found in [5]. The standard has identified eight operating scenarios for WBAN.

- Implant to Implant.
- Implant to Body Surface.
- Implant to External.
- Body Surface to Body Surface (Line-of-Sight (LOS)).
- Body Surface to Body Surface (Non Line-of-Sight (NLOS)).
- Body Surface to External (LOS).
- Body Surface to External (NLOS).

A WBAN can be used for many applications, such as physiological signal monitoring in health care environments, personnel entertainment applications and industrial communication applications for monitoring worker health conditions in safety critical environments. Hence a WBAN should be able to support a variety of data rates from a few bps to several Mbps. With recent advancements in data sensing technologies, the amount of data gathered by sensors has increased dramatically. This increases the demand for high data rate systems to transfer data. For example a 128-channel neural recording system requires a real-time wireless data transmission up to 10 Mbps [6]. Hence, a WBAN should be able to support high data rate communication. Sensor nodes used in either implantable or wearable WBAN applications are battery powered devices. Hence, power efficient operation is a critical aspect of the devices involved in WBAN communication. Furthermore, these implantable and wearable sensor nodes should have a small form factor. Since WBAN sensor nodes operate at a close proximity to the human body, it should operate within various regulations applied for Specific Absorption Rate

(SAR). Hence, transmit power control is important in wireless technologies used for WBAN applications. Basic requirements of a WBAN are listed below [7, 8];

- Support of scalable data rates
- Low power consumption.
- Small form factor.
- Controllable transmit power.
- Ability to prioritise data transmission of crucial signals.
- Secure data transmission.
- Coexistence with other wireless technologies.
- Ability to operate in multi user environments.

A typical WBAN uses a three- tier network structure as shown in Fig. 1.1. Sensor nodes and gateway nodes communicate using short range wireless communication mechanisms. Gateway nodes can choose to communicate with a coordinator node either via a short range wireless communication link or a long range wireless communication link. A Coordinator node forwards data to the internet where data can be transferred to a remote data base. Sensor nodes are connected to a gateway node in a star topology, while several gateway nodes can be connected to a coordinator node using the same topology. Sensor nodes are always attached to the body as either implant devices or wearable devices. Gateway nodes may not be attached to the body; hence, they are not power restricted like sensor nodes. Gateway nodes can communicate with coordinator nodes either using short range Wireless Personnel Area Networks (WPAN) or long range Wireless Local Area Networks (WLAN). WPAN has a range of 10 m while WLAN expands for more than 100 m.

WBANs are used in both medical and non-medical applications. Wireless Electrocardiogram (ECG) monitoring systems and wireless neural recording systems are examples of medical applications that can be implemented using WBAN techniques. WBANs can also be used for non-medical applications such as gaming and smart home control [9]. Several key components can be identified in a WBAN system for healthcare monitoring applications. *Sensor nodes* are either implantable or on-body devices that transmit vital physiological information, such as ECG, Electroencephalogram (EEG) and body temperature to an outside node. A *coordinator node* or a *router node* is used to collect and route the information sent by a sensor node and forward this information to a computer based application for interpretation. Figure 1.2 illustrates the key components of a WBAN.

A WBAN used for healthcare monitoring inherits several key requirements. An implanted or on-body sensor node is battery powered. Especially in the implantable case, human intervention in replacing the batteries should be kept at a minimum level, since it might involve surgical procedures. Hence a WBAN sensor node should consume low power. Low power transmission of signals limits the communication range (usually 0.1–2 m). As a result, an optimized low complexity MAC protocol should be used in WBANs so that it would enhance the low power operation of the sensor node.

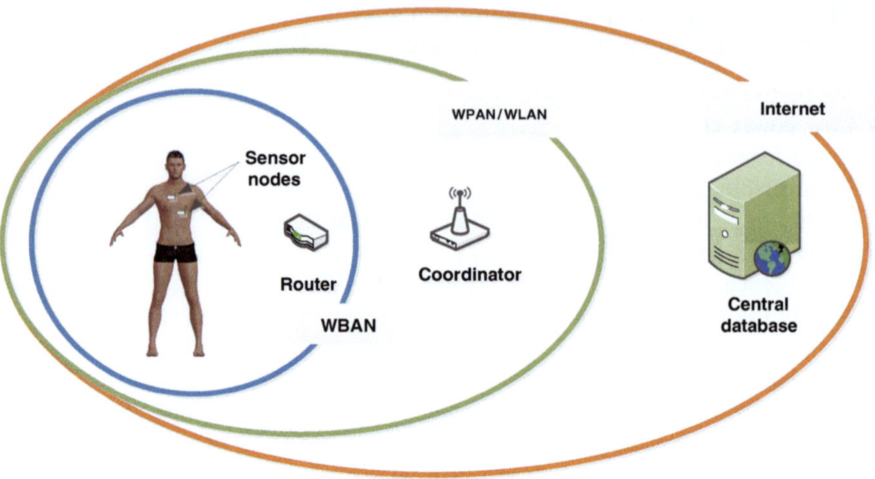

Fig. 1.1 Three-tier communication topology of a WBAN

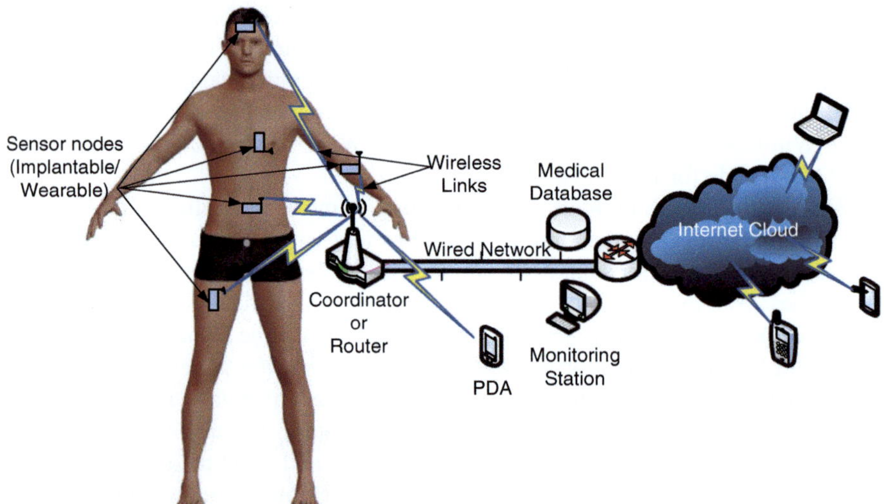

Fig. 1.2 Key components of a WBAN

A WBAN network structure consists of several tiers of interconnecting networks. The work presented in this book pays attention to the communication between sensor nodes and an immediate parent node of the sensor nodes, which can either be a central coordinator or a gateway router. This communication is named as sensor tier communication hereafter. Typically, short-range wireless communication of less than 2 m is employed in the sensor tier. Sensor tier communication is characterized by following features:

- Sensor nodes are connected to the gateway in a star topology.
- Sensor nodes have limited processing capabilities and very stringent requirements on power consumption.
- Unlike sensor nodes, gateway nodes are allowed to have higher processing power and higher battery power.
- Communication is mostly one directional from sensor nodes to a gateway node.
- Communication from the gateway node to sensor nodes consists mainly of network information and feedback.

A WBAN differs from a general Wireless Sensor Network (WSN) application because of its specific requirements. Differences between a WBAN and a more generic WSN are listed in Table 1.1. WBAN applications, such as microelectronic arrays and neural recording systems, use multi-channel monitoring, which drastically increases the amount of data that needs to be transmitted simultaneously. Wireless Capsule Endoscopy (WCE) is another type of WBAN devices that requires high data rates for high resolution video transmission. Thus, there is a demand for high data rate transmission of medical data. For example, a 128-channel neural recording system with eight bit sampling requires a data rate in excess of 10 Mbps [6]. Use of wired connections for data transmission is not feasible at all times. It restricts the movement of the patient and involves painful surgical procedures (for example in WCE). Basic requirements of a WBAN are listed below.

1. Limited transmission range (<0.01–2 m).
2. Extremely low power consumption in sleep mode (0.1–0.5 mW) for each device for longer battery life.
3. Support of scalable data rate ranging from 1 kbps to several Mbps.
4. Quality of Service (QoS) support for better handling of critical physiological signals.
5. Low latency over a multi-hop network.
6. Small form factor and light weight devices.

1.2 Physical Layer Wireless Technologies Used in WBAN Applications

There are several wireless technologies currently considered for data communication in WBAN applications. This section gives a brief introduction to some of these important wireless technologies.

Table 1.1 Differences between a WBAN and a WSN

Property	WBAN	WSN
Sensor position	Located in or on a human body or at a close proximity to a human body	Deployed over a large area
Topology	Typically comprises of multiple sensor nodes and one central receiving node (gateway node). All the sensor nodes will communicate directly with the gateway node forming a star topology	Sensors are connected based on mesh-topology, where multiple hops are supported. Each sensor in a WSN can act as a router node
Nature of data	Data from physiological signals is periodic and signals are transmitted at a fixed interval. For example, the transmission frequency of a temperature sensor can be once every minute [10]	The nature of data depends on the application. The transmission interval for WSN is irregular
Redundancy	Because of the limited space and limited sensor locations for measuring the physiological signals on the human body, only one sensor exists for measuring each physiological signal. There is no redundancy that allows for node failure in WBAN	More than one sensor can be deployed in WSN to allow for redundancy, Especially in areas where data is critical or where sensors are inaccessible
Mobility	Human body movement is unpredictable. Body movements such as bending down or swinging arms will affect the channel condition of the nodes. The interference level for WBAN systems is also unpredictable due to mobility. The level of interference will increase, when two or more users move towards each other	Nodes for WSN are typically stationary, making channel conditions more predictable
Data collection	Multiple receivers (e.g. PDAs carried by doctors and nurses) are used in WBAN systems to collect data from sensor nodes	Focuses on best-effort data collection at the central database

1.2.1 Zigbee

The Zigbee standard defines the network, security and application layer on top of the IEEE 802.15.4 standard [11], which incorporates the physical and MAC layers [12]. The physical layer of the IEEE 802.15.4 standard supports several frequency bands for data communication. It supports one channel of 20 kbps in 868 MHz band, 10 channels of 40 kbps each in 915 MHz and 16 channels of 250 kbps each in 2.4 GHz band. The MAC layer of the IEEE 802.15.4 standard is based on

Carrier Sense Multiple Access with Collision Avoidance (CSMA/CA) for media access.

Zigbee network topology defines three types of nodes: end-devices, router nodes and coordinator nodes. A Zigbee coordinator node initiates the network and manages network resources. Zigbee router nodes enable multi-hop communication between the devices in a network. Zigbee's end-devices communicate with parent nodes (router nodes or coordinator nodes) and operate with minimal functionality in order to reduce the power consumption.

The Zigbee Alliance acts as the main body that provides application profiles for Zigbee based applications. Zigbee based healthcare applications are intended to be used in non-invasive healthcare platforms. MICAZ by Crossbow [13] is an example of a commercial hardware platform that supports Zigbee communication.

Zigbee technology has several drawbacks for healthcare applications. It operates in the 2.4 GHz unlicensed industrial, scientific and medical (ISM) band alongside with WLANs and Bluetooth making the 2.4 GHz band more crowded. The power consumption of a Zigbee based sensor node is considerably high. For example, the Chipcon IC (CC2420), which is a commercially available transceiver has a current consumption of 17.4 mA in transmit mode and 19.7 mA in receive mode [14].

1.2.2 Wireless Local Area Networks

Wireless Local Area Networks (WLAN) operate based on the physical and MAC layer protocols developed in the IEEE 802.11 standard. Different versions of the IEEE 802.11 standards use different physical layer communication mechanisms. For example, the IEEE 802.11 g standard uses Orthogonal Frequency Division Multiplexing (OFDM) while the IEEE 802.11b standard uses Direct Sequence Spread Spectrum (DSSS) for physical layer communication. Even though WLAN standards are able to cater for the high data rate requirement of WBAN applications, it is rarely used in WBAN applications because of its large power consumption. For example, the most recent implementations of WLAN transmitters consume around 82 mW of power [15].

1.2.3 Medical Implant Communication Services

Medical Implant Communication Services (MICS) band uses the 401–406 MHz frequency band allocated by the Federal Communications Commission (FCC) in order to transmit data from an implanted device to an outside controller [16]. Ten channels with 300 kHz bandwidth are allocated for communication within this band. The transmit power of the communication devices that uses the MICS band is limited to −16 dBm by the FCC regulations. The use of low transmission frequency in MICS band results in low propagation loss within an implant communication environment. The regulations require MICS transceivers to use interference mitigation techniques in order to prevent interference with other radio services operating within the same frequency band. MICS devices use Listen-Before-Talk (LBT) technique in order to listen to the wireless channel before starting communication. If the channel is busy, an MICS transceiver uses Adaptive Frequency Agile (AFA) technique in order to switch into another channel. However, use of MICS band is limited to low data rate applications and it cannot be used for WBAN applications that require high data rates due to its bandwidth limitations.

1.2.4 Bluetooth

Bluetooth operates in the 2.4 GHz ISM band and uses Frequency Hopping Spread Spectrum (FHSS) in order to access the physical medium [17]. Bluetooth bandwidth spans from 2402 to 2480 MHz over 79 channels with 1 MHz channel bandwidth. It communicates based on piconet network topology, where each device in a piconet has the ability to communicate with seven other devices in the same piconet. Low energy Bluetooth technology [18] was introduced in 2009 with the intention of reducing the power consumption in Bluetooth devices. Like the Zigbee technology, Bluetooth also suffers from the interference in the 2.4 GHz band. It also lacks the scalability in terms of data rate and number of supported devices.

1.2.5 Ultra-Wideband

History of UWB communication goes back to the Hertizian spark gap experiments conducted in 1880. Shannon's experiments in 1948 highlighted the advantages of spread spectrum communication systems. In 1960s UWB attracted attention within the scientific community for radar applications. Early UWB devices consumed large amount of power; hence UWB technology was not considered for data communication applications. Emergence of semiconductor devices in the latter half of the twentieth century created the possibility of low power UWB signal generation techniques. In 2002, Federal Communications Commission (FCC) created the first report that approved UWB communication for commercial use [19]. Under this report UWB is defined as signals having a fractional bandwidth (−10 dB bandwidth) of more than 20 %, or a bandwidth of at least 500 MHz. FCC has applied stringent power requirements on UWB transmission. It allows peak power limit of 0 dBm and average power limit of −41.3 dBm/MHz. UWB is allowed to operate in both 0–960 MHz and 3.1–10.6 GHz bands. In 2005 FCC updated its

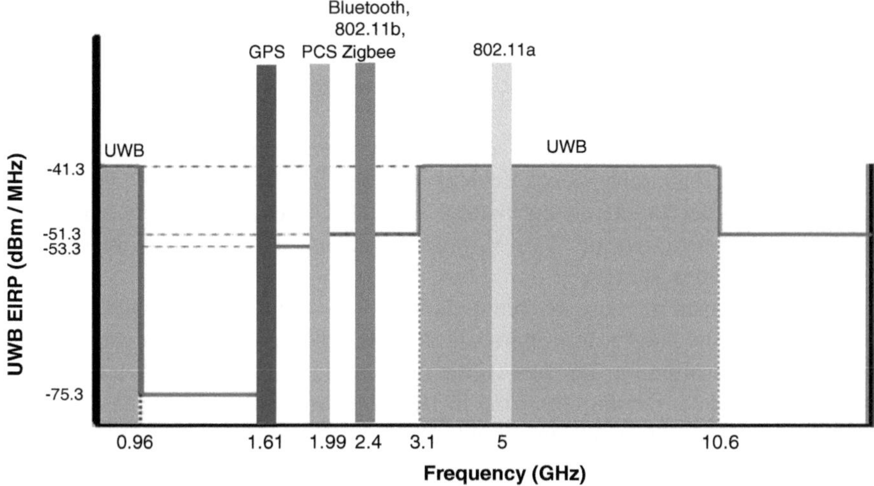

Fig. 1.3 Transmit spectrums for UWB and other wireless technologies

regulations on UWB transmit power allowing gated UWB transmission systems to transmit at higher peak powers [20]. In March 2007, an international standard for UWB communication was approved by the International Organization for Standardization (ISO) based on the Wi-Media UWB common radio platform [21, 22]. Figure 1.3 depicts the frequency spectrum of UWB transmission together with spectrums of other existing wireless technologies.

UWB communication systems can be divided into two major categories; Impulse Radio-Ultra-Wideband (IR-UWB) and Multi Carrier-Ultra-Wideband (MC-UWB). MC-UWB uses multiple sub carriers to transmit data using Orthogonal Frequency Division Multiplexing (OFDM). This technique is used by the Wi-Media alliance for wireless multimedia transmission. MC-UWB technique consumes large amount of power due to complex signal processing involved in OFDM based transceivers. For example, the Wi-Media chipset by Aleron consumes around 300 mW of power [23]; hence, it is not suitable for power stringent WBAN applications.

IR-UWB systems transmit short pulses to transmit data. Pulsed nature of UWB transmitters enables the use of simpler modulation schemes such as Pulse Position Modulation (PPM) and On-Off-Keying (OOK). Simpler modulation schemes enable less complex hardware systems implementing IR-UWB communication systems and reduce the power consumption significantly. These are among many advantages provided by the IR-UWB communication systems, making it a suitable candidate for battery powered WBAN applications. Some of the major advantages provided by the IR-UWB communication for WBAN applications are discussed in the following section.

1.3 IR-UWB WBAN System and Advantages

(1) Low power consumption of IR-UWB transmitters

WBAN devices are considered as battery powered devices. Hence, the power consumption of data transmission devices involved in a WBAN should be kept at a minimum in order to extend the battery life. This is especially very critical for implantable applications of WBAN, since replacing a device or a battery will involve an invasive surgery.

IR-UWB transmitters use discrete pulses in order to transmit data [24], whereas traditional narrow band transmitters use data modulated continuous wave signals for wireless transmission. Because of the discrete pulse transmission, a significant portion of the data transmission time in IR-UWB transmitters consists of a silent period. As a result, the electronic components involved in pulse generation can be operated at a low power mode. In contrast, traditional narrow band transmitters operate continuously throughout the data transmission period for most of modulation schemes. This difference of data mapping principal results in a significant reduction in the power consumption UWB based wireless technologies for long operation periods.

Implementation of an IR-UWB transmitter involves very few Radio Frequency (RF) components compared to continuous wave transmitters. In fact, all digital realizations of IR-UWB transmitters are achievable with the aid of state-of-the-art Complementary Metal Oxide Semiconductor (CMOS) technology [25]. In contrast, traditional narrow band transmitters utilize high power consuming RF and analog components, such as RF Power Amplifiers (PA) and analog Phase Locked Loops (PLL), extensively due to the nature of the signal generation [26].

Furthermore, because of the easier data mapping in IR-UWB transmitter, complex modulation schemes are not required for IR-UWB communication systems. This feature enhances the power savings significantly. Hence, IR-UWB communication may provide a significant advantage over traditional narrow band transmitters for power intensive WBAN applications.

(2) High data rate capability

IR-UWB radios map the data bits into very short (nano second duration) pulses. This method implies a carrier-less data transmission scheme, where short pulses represent a signal with a signal power that is spread in a large bandwidth in the frequency domain. According to Shannon's capacity theorem, the data rate capacity of a channel is linearly proportional to its channel bandwidth and logarithmically proportional to increase in the Signal to Noise Ratio (SNR) of the channel. This means that the IR-UWB signals are capable of delivering higher data rates, using the high bandwidth property. A continuous wave based narrow band signal has to operate at much higher frequencies in order to transmit at the same data rates [27]. The use of higher frequencies in narrow band signals leads to higher attenuation, which has to be compensated by increasing the transmit power.

Hence, an IR-UWB transmission system is capable of achieving higher data rates while operating at low power, which makes it an ideal candidate for power intensive WBAN applications that demand high data rates, such as wireless capsule endoscopy systems [28, 29] and neural recording systems [6].

(3) Small form factor

Small size is an essential property for implantable and wearable WBAN sensor nodes. IR-UWB transmitters can be manufactured with only a few electronic components: hence the design space required is minimal. This is an advantageous property that makes IR-UWB a suitable candidate for WBAN sensor nodes.

(4) Susceptibility to multipath interference

IR-UWB uses finite resolution pulses in order to represent data bits. Unlike in the case of continuous wave signals where multipath components always overlap with time domain signals at the receiver end, the multipath arrivals of the IR-UWB signals can be easily resolved and avoided at the receiver end because of the low probability of a multipath component overlapping with the received narrow pulse in the time domain [30, 31]. This is a very useful feature in IR-UWB when it is operating around the body where the presence of multipath components can be high.

In spite of these advantages, there are some drawbacks in IR-UWB technology that should be overcome for WBAN applications. These disadvantages are listed below:

(1) Complexity of the IR-UWB receiver architecture

IR-UWB signals use narrow pulses to transmit data and the transmitted signal power is regulated to be very low in order to prevent interference to other systems. An IR-UWB receiver has to be capable of detecting these low power narrow pulses. This requires the use of high speed Analog to Digital Converters (ADC) and extensive amplification of the received signals at IR-UWB receiver front-end. This makes the IR-UWB receiver to be complex in design and results in increased power consumption. This is a major drawback in IR-UWB systems that should be overcome in order to use IR-UWB for power intensive WBAN applications.

(2) Susceptibility to interference from other wireless transmission systems

Unlike in the case of carrier based systems, IR-UWB signal power is spread across a wide bandwidth. Hence it is susceptible to interference from all the systems operating within the IR-UWB signal bandwidth. The signal processing involved in the reception of carrier based signals has to consider only the interference rejection in that particular carrier frequency, whereas for IR-UWB systems, the signal processing at the receiver end should consider interference mitigation for the whole signal bandwidth. This problem can be overcome by choosing a suitable operational bandwidth with minimum interference for IR-UWB communication. Figure 1.4

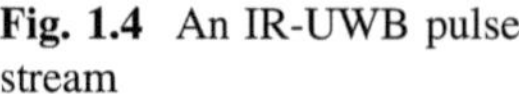

Fig. 1.4 An IR-UWB pulse stream

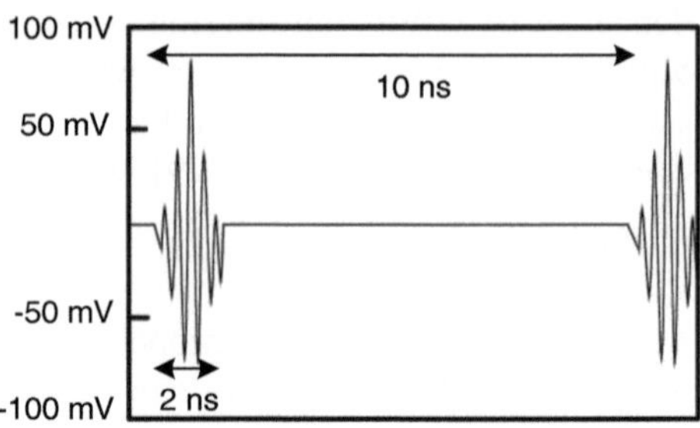

depicts an IR-UWB pulse stream generated by an IR-UWB transmitter. This pulse stream consists of IR-UWB pulses with a pulse width of 2 ns and a Pulse Repetitive Frequency (PRF) of 100 MHz.

1.4 Comparison of Wireless Technologies Used for WBAN

This section compares the candidate wireless technologies that can be used in WBAN applications in terms of data rate capability, susceptibility to interference, power consumption and form factor. Table 1.2 depicts some of the wireless technologies used in WBAN applications. Out of the existing wireless physical layer technologies, UWB and WLAN standards are able to cater for the high data rate requirement of WBAN applications such as neural recording and WCE. However, WLAN is rarely used in WBAN applications because of its large power consumption. MICS band can only be used for low data rate WBAN applications due to its limited bandwidth capabilities.

Zigbee, Bluetooth and WLAN operate in the 2.4 GHz unlicensed ISM band; hence create interference issues to each other [32, 33]. UWB frequency spectrum is affected by the interference due to the operation of WLAN devices in the 5 GHz band. However, it is possible to choose the operational bandwidth of UWB from a wide spectrum that ranges from 3.1–10 GHz. Hence, the GHz interference can be avoided if a sub-band of UWB spectrum is used for UWB communication. The MICS band has a dedicated spectrumfor data communication; hence, it is subjected to minimum interference from other wireless technologies.

Low power consumption and small form factor are important aspects of a wireless technology that can be used in WBAN applications. In order to assess these capabilities of a particular wireless technology, it is important to analyze some of the wireless sensor platforms that have been developed based on different wireless technologies. Table 1.3 depicts some of the available WBAN platforms that are commonly considered for WBAN applications. These devices operate using a low supply voltage ranging from 2–3 V. From the available narrowband sensor platforms, Microsemi (formerly Zarlink) platform provides a Complementary Metal

Table 1.2 Candidate wireless technologies for WBAN communication

Properties	Wireless technology					
	Zigbee	WLAN		MICS	Bluetooth	UWB
Frequency	2.4 GHz	2.4 GHz	5 GHz	401–406 MHz	2.4 GHz	3.1–10.6 GHz
Transmit power	0 dBm	10–30 dBm	10–30 dBm	−16 dBm	0 dBm	−41.3 dBm/ MHz
Number of channels	16	13	23	10	10	–
Channel bandwidth	2 MHz	22 MHz	20 or 40 MHz	300 kHz	1 MHz	≥500 MHz
Data rate	250 kbps	11 Mbps	54 Mbps	200–800 kbps	1 Mbps	850 kbps up to 20 Mbps
Range	0–10 m	0–100 m	0–100 m	0–10 m	0–10 m	2 m

Oxide Semiconductor (CMOS) based Integrated Circuit (IC) transceiver with the lowest power consumption based on the MICS and 433 MHz ISM bands for WBAN applications. This IC is used in the Given Imaging's PillCam WCE devices for low power narrow band based implant communication [34]. The MICA2DOT sensor platform provides a full hardware implementation on a small sensor platform. However, the power consumption of the transmitter is considerably high compared to that of the Microsemi's narrow band system. An implementation of a small wearable pulse wave monitoring system that uses a Bluetooth based transceiver is presented in [35]. The total current consumption of the systems is estimated to be 51 mA, inclusive of the current consumption of the Bluetooth transceiver, which is estimated to be 21 mA with an operating voltage of 3.3 V. The power consumption in a Zigbee and 2.4 GHz ISM band based sensor nodes are considerably high compared to other sensor node designs. The comparison in Table 1.3 shows that the if a sensor node is designed based on UWB utilizing mainly a transmitter and minimizing/eliminating the use of a receiver, it will perform better than the narrowband based systems in terms of power consumption, form factor and data rate.

It can be concluded that the UWB presents some unique benefits over other wireless technologies in the design of WBAN sensor nodes including the low power requirements of UWB transmitter, high data rate capability, low form factor and reasonably uncomplicated circuit design. In terms of interference rejection, UWB spectrum provides a large bandwidth; hence, a sub-band of UWB can be selected for a particular application such that the interference from other bands is minimized. Furthermore, IR-UWB is preferred over MC-UWB because of the possibility of low complexity and low power consuming hardware implementation. IR-UWB is referred to as UWB in the remainder of this book unless mentioned otherwise.

Table 1.3 Sensor platforms for WBAN applications

Sensor	Company	Wireless technology	Frequency	Data rate	Physical dimension	Power/Current	
						Tx.	Rx.
UWB based	Ref. [36]	UWB	3.5–4.5 GHz	10 Mbps	27 × 25 × 1.5 mm (board)	8 mW	–
	Ref. [37]	UWB – Tx., ISM- Rx.	Tx.- 3.5–4.5 GHz, Rx.- 433 MHz	Tx. -5 Mbps Rx.- 19.2 kbps	30 × 25 × 0.5 mm (board)	3 mW	10 mW
	Ref. [28]	UWB	3.1–10.6 GHz	10Mbps	3 × 4 mm^2 (IC) 5 cm (board length)	0.35 mW	62 mW at 10 Mbps
Mica2 (MPR400)	Crossbow [13]	ISM (Proprietary)	868/916 MHz	38.4 kbps	58 × 32 × .7 mm (board)	27 mA	10 mA
MicAz	Crossbow [13]	Zigbee	2.4 GHz	250 kbps	58 × 32 × .7 mm (board)	17.4 mA	19.7 mA
Mica2DOT	Crossbow [13]	ISM (Proprietary)	433 MHz	38.4 kbps	25 × 6 mm^2 (board)	25 mA	8 mA
CC1010	TI [38]	Narrow band (Proprietary)	300–1000 MHz	76.8 kbps	12 × 12 mm^2 (IC)	26.6 mA	11.9 mA
CC2400	TI [38]	ISM (Proprietary)	2.4 GHz	1 Mbps	7.1 × 7.1 mm2 (IC)	19 mA	23 mA
MICS based	Microsemi—ZL70250 (Formerly Zarlink) [39] Ref. [40]	MICS	402–405 MHz, 433 MHz ISM	800 kbps	7 × 7 mm^2 (IC)	5 mA under continuous TX/RX operation	
		MICS	402–405 MHz	8 kbps	–	25 mA	7.5 mA
Bluetooth based	KK-22 [35]	Bluetooth	2.4 GHz	115 kbps	18 mm^2 (board)	21 mA under continuous TX/RX operation	

1.5 Scope of the Book

This book focuses on several important areas regarding WBAN and IR-UWB communication that are described below;

(1) Hardware platform development for IR-UWB based WBAN communication

This book thoroughly discusses several hardware design techniques that can be used in the development of IR-UWB based hardware platforms that include IR-UWB transceiver design techniques and full sensor node implementations. This book also presents the development of a unique sensor node design that uses an IR-UWB transmitter for data transmission and a 433 MHz ISM band receiver for data reception. Furthermore, development of a dual band coordinator node that facilitates the data communication of multiple sensor nodes is presented. Various properties of IR-UWB pulses such as rise time, pulse width and PRF, are analyzed in detail in order to develop an IR-UWB transmitter with optimum performance.

(2) MAC protocols for IR-UWB based WBANs

MAC protocol plays a key role in facilitating reliable and power efficient communication between multiple sensor nodes. This book discusses various MAC protocols that are available in the literature paying attention to their critical aspects, such as power efficiency, throughput capability and data transmission delay. This book also presents a UWB MAC protocol that provides efficient data transmission in WBANs applications. This MAC protocol uses a beacon enabled super frame structure in order to schedule the data transmissions of sensor nodes; hence reduces the multiple access interference in the network. Furthermore, it is designed to dynamically control the Pulses Per Bit (PPB) value used for UWB data communication using control messages sent via the narrow band feedback path. This leads to dynamic BER and power control at the sensor nodes, which helps to improve the reliability of communication and power efficiency of sensor nodes under dynamic channel conditions. A simulation platform developed using the Opnet modeler [41], which is a commercially available network simulation software, is presented. Important properties of the UWB communication system, such as physical layer pulse based UWB transmission, multipath and fading properties of IR-UWB and WBAN channel models, and multiple user interference, are incorporated into this simulation platform. Main intention of these simulation-based studies is to investigate the feasibility of the UWB communication method before going into hardware implementation. It also provides a mean of analyzing the performance of the UWB MAC protocol in an environment where a large number of sensor nodes are involved in communication.

(3) Implementation and experimental evaluation of a UWB MAC protocol in hardware platforms

This book discusses the implementation considerations of UWB MAC protocol spaying attentions to features, such as synchronization of IR-UWB signals, data packet structures and dynamic configuration of sensor nodes according to the change in propagation channel conditions. Performance of the MAC protocol isalso analyzed in terms of important performance indicators, such as Bit Error Rate (BER) delay and power consumption of the sensor nodes.

(4) Analysis of the electromagnetic effects of UWB communication for implant applications

High data rate implant communication is one of the lucrative future directions for IR-UWB communication. This book presents studiesof the electromagnetic effects of IR-UWB based implant communication systems, such as the variation of Specific Absorption Rate (SAR) and tissue temperature increase, through finite element based simulations, which successfully show the feasibility of IR-UWB communication for implant devices.

References

1. http://www.who.int/topics/ageing/en/ (2013)
2. M.R. Yuce, J. Khan, *Wireless Body Area Networks: Technology, Implementation and Applications* (Pan Stanford Publishing, 2011) ISBN 978-981-431-6712, 2011
3. P.S. Hall, Y. Hao, K. Ito, Guest editorial for the special issue on antennas and propagation on body-centric wireless communications. IEEE Trans. Antennas Propag. **57**(4), 834–836 (2009)
4. http://www.ieee802.org/15/pub/TG6.html (2014)
5. The IEEE 804.15.6 Standard (2012) Wireless body area networks
6. M. Chae, Z. Yang, M.R. Yuce, L. Hoang, W. Liu, A 128-channel 6 mW wireless neural recording IC with spike feature extraction and UWB transmitter. IEEE Trans. Neural Syst. Rehabil. Eng. **17**(4), 312–321 (2009)
7. L. Huan-Bang, R. Kohno, Introduction of SG-BAN in IEEE 802.15 with related discussion. In: *IEEE International Conference on Ultra-Wideband,* pp. 134–139, Sept 2007
8. M.R. Yuce, Implementation of wireless body area networks for healthcare systems. Sens. Actuators, A **162**, 116–129 (2010)
9. W. Tiexiang, W. Lei, G. Jia, H. Bangyu, A 3-D acceleration-based control algorithm for interactive gaming using a head-worn wireless device. In: 3rd *International Conference on Bioinformatics and Biomedical Engineering,* pp. 1–3, 2009
10. K. Takizawa, L. Huan-Bang, K. Hamaguchi, R. Kohno, Wireless patient monitoring using IEEE 802.15.4a WPAN. In: *IEEE International Conference on Ultra-Wideband,* pp. 235–240, 2007
11. IEEE-802. Part 15.4: wireless medium access control (MAC) and physical layer (PHY) specifications for low-rate wireless personal area networks (LR-WPANs). Standard, IEEE, 15 April 2006
12. http://www.zigbee.org/ (2014)
13. http://www.xbow.com/ (2014)
14. http://focus.ti.com/docs/prod/folders/print/cc2420.html (2014)
15. P. Madoglio, A. Ravi, H. Xu, K. Chandrashekar, M. Verhelst, S. Pellerano, L. Cuellar, M. Aguirre, M. Sajadieh, O. Degani, H. Lakdawala, Y. Palaskas, A 20 dBm 2.4 GHz digital out

phasing transmitter for WLAN application in 32 nm CMOS. In: *IEEE International Solid-State Circuits Conference Digest of Technical Papers*, pp.168,170, 19–23 Feb 2012

16. FCC Rules and regulations, MICS band plan, Part 95, Jan 2003
17. http://www.bluetooth.com/Pages/Bluetooth-Home.aspx (2013)
18. http://www.bluetooth.com/Pages/Bluetooth-Smart.aspx (2013)
19. FCC 02-48 (First Report and Order) (2002)
20. FCC 05-58: Petition for waiver of the part 15 UWB regulations. Filed by the Multi-band OFDM Alliance Special Interest Group, ET Docket 04-352, 11, March 2005
21. ISO/IEC 26907:2007—Information technology—telecommunications and information exchange between systems—high rate ultra wideband PHY and MAC standard (2007)
22. http://www.wimedia.org/ (2013)
23. http://www.alereon.com/products/chipsets/ (2013)
24. M.R. Yuce, H.C. Keong, M. Chae, Wideband communication for implantable and wearable systems. IEEE Trans. Microw Theory Tech. **57**(2), 2597–2604 (2009)
25. Y. Park, D.D. Wentzloff, An all-digital 12 pJ/pulse IR-UWB transmitter synthesized from a standard cell library. IEEE J. Solid-State Circuits **46**(5), 1147,1157 (2011)
26. A.C.W. Wong, M. Dawkins, G. Devita, N. Kasparidis, A. Katsiamis, O. King, F. Lauria, J. Schiff, A.J. Burdett, A 1 V 5 mA multimode IEEE 802.15.6/bluetooth low-energy WBAN transceiver for biotelemetry applications. IEEE J. Solid-State Circuits **48**(1), 186, 198 (2013)
27. K. Okada, N. Li, K. Matsushita, K. Bunsen, R. Murakami, A. Musa, T. Sato, H. Asada, N. Takayama, S. Ito, W. Chaivipas, R. Minami, T. Yamaguchi, Y. Takeuchi, H. Yamagishi, M. Noda, A. Matsuzawa, A 60-GHz 16QAM/8PSK/QPSK/BPSK direct-conversion transceiver for IEEE802.15.3c. IEEE J. Solid-State Circuits **46**(12), 2988, 3004 (2011)
28. Y. Gao, Y. Zheng, S. Diao, W. Toh, C. Ang, M. Je, C. Heng, Low-power ultrawideband wireless telemetry transceiver for medical sensor applications. IEEE Trans. Biomed. Eng. **58**(3), 768,772 (2011)
29. M.R.Yuce, T. Dissanayake, Easy-to-swallow wireless telemetry. IEEE Microwave Mag. **13**(6), 90–101 (2012)
30. Y. Zhao, L. Wang, J.-F.Frigon, C. Nerguizian, K. Wu, R.G. Bosisio, UWB positioning using six-port technology and a learning machine. In: *IEEE Mediterranean Electrotechnical Conference*, pp. 352–355, 16–19 May 2006
31. G. Kail, K. Witrisal, F. Hlawatsch, Direction-resolved estimation of multipath parameters for UWB channels: A partially collapsed Gibbs sampler method. In: *IEEE International Conference on Acoustics, Speech and Signal Processing*, pp. 3484–3487, 22–27 May 2011
32. H. Hongwei, X. Youzhi, C. C. Bilen, and Z. Hongke, Coexistence issues of 2.4ghz sensor networks with other rf devices at home. In: *International Conference on Sensor Technologies and Applications*, pp. 200–205, June 2009
33. A. Mathew, N. Chandrababu, K. Elleithy, S. Rizvi, IEEE 802.11 & bluetooth interference: simulation and coexistence. In: *Seventh Annual Communication Networks and Services Research Conference*, pp. 217–223, May 2009
34. http://www.givenimaging.com/en-us/Innovative-Solutions/Capsule-Endoscopy/Pillcam-SB/Pages/default.aspx (2013)
35. K. Sonoda, Y. Kishida, T. Tanaka, K. Kanda, T. Fujita, K. Maenaka, and K. Higuchi, Wearable photoplethysmographic sensor system with PSoC microcontroller. In: *Fifth International Conference on Emerging Trends in Engineering and Technology (ICETET)*, pp. 61–65, 2012
36. H.C. Keong, K.M. Thotahewa, M.R. Yuce, Transmit-only ultra wide band (UWB) body sensors and collision analysis. IEEE Sens. J. **13**, 1949–1958 (2013)
37. K.M. Thotahewa, J-M.Redoute, M.R. Yuce, Implementation of a dual band body sensor node. In: *IEEE MTT-S International Microwave Workshop Series on RF and Wireless Technologies for Biomedical and Healthcare (IMWS- Bio2013)*, 2013

38. http://www.ti.com/ (2014)
39. http://www.microsemi.com/ (2014)
40. M.R. Yuce et al., Wireless body sensor network using medical implant band. J. Med. Syst. **31**, 467–474 (2007)
41. http://www.opnet.com/ (2014)

Chapter 2
MAC Protocols for UWB-Based WBAN Applications

Abstract Wireless Body Area Network (WBAN) is a networking concept that has evolved with the idea of monitoring vital physiological signals from low-power and miniaturized in-body or on-body sensors. In a WBAN, data collected from the sensor nodes are transferred to a remote node via a wireless medium, where the data is forwarded to a higher layer application to be interpreted. A WBAN system might require both real time and periodic data transfer. Since WBAN sensor nodes are battery powered, they should be low-power devices. The sensor tier communication of a WBAN involves the co-existence of WBAN hardware and Medium Access Control (MAC) protocol that enable the efficient communication of sensor data. The main focus of this chapter is to investigate key aspects of MAC protocols used in WBAN systems focusing on UWB as the wireless technology. This chapter also discusses the wireless technologies used for WBAN applications, paying attention to their ability to cater to the need of high data rate while operating at a low power. Key advantages of Ultra-wide band (UWB) over the other wireless technologies for WBAN applications are highlighted herein.

Keywords UWB · MAC · Algorithm · Packet formats · IEEE 802. 15. 6 · IEEE 802. 15. 4a · Transmit-only UWB · Dual-band

2.1 Introduction

The basic requirement of wireless healthcare monitoring systems is to send physiological signals acquired from implantable or on-body sensor nodes to a remote location. Low-power consumption is required for wireless healthcare monitoring systems since most medical sensor nodes are battery powered. The emergence of new technologies in measuring physiological signals has increased the demand for high data rate transmission systems. UWB is a suitable wireless technology to achieve high data rates while keeping power consumption and form factors small. The main drawback of the UWB technology is its receiver

K. M. S. Thotahewa et al., *Ultra Wideband Wireless Body Area Networks*, 19
DOI: 10.1007/978-3-319-05287-8_2,

complexity. Due to the short pulse width and low power level of the transmitted signal, the front-end circuitry of an UWB receiver is complex in design and has high power consumption [1]. Synchronization of the IR-UWB pulses at receive stage using low power front end circuitry is one of the major problems that restricts the use of IR-UWB receivers for implant applications.

MAC protocols for UWB systems govern the multiple access of the UWB channel. The MAC protocols for UWB systems have to be designed in a way such that they enhance the advantages provided by the UWB signals and overcome the drawbacks such as high receiver complexity [2]. In general, MAC protocols based on carrier sensing and Clear Channel Assessment (CCA) are not appropriate for UWB based MAC protocols, because it is extremely difficult to assess the channel condition of a wideband UWB channel that uses narrow pulses to transmit data. CCA for IR-UWB cannot be implemented using a peak detector, matched filter or correlation method [3]. A frequency domain method to implement CCA for IR-UWB signal is proposed in [3]. This method requires a large number of narrowband filters and energy detectors. The proposed circuit is designed for the detection of IR-UWB signals spread across the entire 7.5 GHz band. It is not suitable for channelized UWB systems where only a sub-band of UWB is utilised. In a channelized UWB system, the typical transmission bandwidth is between 500 MHz to 1 GHz. Most of the energy detectors in the CCA circuit will register a false reading when a strong narrowband interferer is present.

The MAC protocols for UWB systems may preferably use a random medium access method or a transmit-only MAC protocol for the multiple access of the UWB channel. This chapter intends to give a critical analysis of the recently published work on UWB MAC protocols that has the potential usage for WBAN applications.

2.2 The IEEE 802.15.6 Standard

The IEEE 802.15.6 standard [4] is the first standard that defines the MAC architecture for in-body and on-body wireless communications. The standard defines the physical layer communication using UWB and other narrow band technologies. The standard recommends the star topology to form a network for the wireless nodes in a WBAN. Multiple access is achieved in the time domain with the aid of a super frame structure. The super frame is divided into equal length time slots, which are allocated to the contending sensor nodes by a central coordinator, which controls the shared access to the wireless medium.

The IEEE 802.15.6 standard supports three communication modes [4]:

1. Beacon mode with super frame boundaries:

The super frame structure is divided by beacons transmitted in the downlink by the coordinator in this communication mode. Several medium access mechanisms are supported for sensor nodes communicating using this mode: Exclusive access, Managed access, Random access and Contention access. Exclusive access and Managed access periods in the super frame are used to provide guaranteed data transfer for sensor nodes with high priority while other two methods provide data transfer for less priority sensor nodes.

2. Non-beacon mode with super frame boundaries:

This communication mode does not use a downlink beacon in order to indicate the super frame boundaries to the sensor nodes. Instead it uses the scheduling of data communication through techniques, such as polling. The coordinator schedules the data transmission of each individual sensor node through polling, such that the data communication from the sensor nodes falls within a super frame structure. This communication mode falls within the Managed access.

3. Non-beacon mode without super frame boundaries:

In this communication mode a pre-defined super frame structure is not used. The data communication occurs through polling or posted allocation where a certain amount of timeslots are allocated by the coordinator node, which can be accessed by any sensor node waiting for data transmission.

The access to the shared medium is provided using various mechanisms [4]:

1. Random access using slotted ALOHA and CSMA/CA.
2. Improvised and unscheduled access mechanism, where the coordinator node send polling and posting commands without pre-reservation or pre-scheduling in a random manner.
3. Scheduled access using polling.

The UWB physical layer (PHY) specifications in the IEEE 802.15.6 standard is used to provide high data rate and low power consuming data transfer using UWB signals. The UWB spectrum in the range of 3.1–10 GHz is divided into eleven channels with a channel bandwidth of 499.2 MHz for each channel. The PHY specifications support both IR-UWB and Frequency Modulation-UWB (FM-UWB). This section will only discuss the specifications for IR-UWB, as it is better suited for WBAN applications because of the possibility of implementing low complexity hardware for IR-UWB transmitters.

The IEEE 802.15.6 standard supports three different modulation schemes for IR-UWB: On-Off Keying (OOK), Differential Binary Phase Shift Keying (DBPSK) and Differential Quadrature Phase Shift Keying (DQPSK). The Physical layer Protocol Data Unit (PPDU) for the IR-UWB based data communication is shown in Fig. 2.1.

The Synchronisation Header (SHR) provides a preamble bit pattern (*Kasami* sequence with a length of 63) which is essential part in the narrow pulse based UWB data transmission. The PHY Header (PHR) provides 24 data fields which are used to indicate communication parameters such as data rate, MAC frame body

Fig. 2.1 The IEEE 802.15.6 standard physical layer protocol data unit (PPDU) for IR-UWB PHY specifications

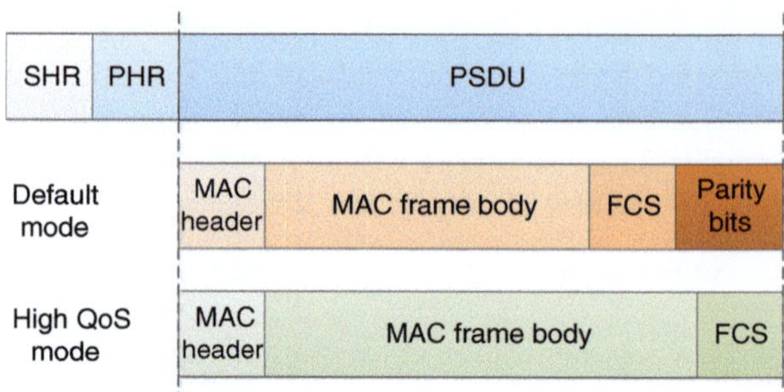

length, pulse type (chirp pulse, chaotic pulse and short pulse) and modulation mode. The IEEE 802.15.6 standard supports also bit interleaving using a modulus interleaver in order to provide robust data transmission by avoiding large sequences of consecutive ones and zeros. Because of the difficulty in CCA for UWB, a random access mechanism based on the slotted ALOHA or a polling based medium access mechanism is recommended for UWB based WBANS in the IEEE 802.15.6 standard.

Drawbacks: although the IEEE 802.15.6 standard defines a robust standard for WBAN applications, it has several drawbacks when it comes to using UWB for WBAN applications. It ignores several key limitations in the implementation of the UWB transceivers. The MAC protocol defined by the IEEE 802.15.6 standard utilises a UWB receiver at the sensor node end. Although the UWB transmitters are relatively less complex, the implementation of the UWB receiver requires power hungry complex circuit design. In addition, the MAC protocol defined in the standard ignores the optimisation of the UWB transmit power control through duty cycling and gated pulse transmission techniques [5, 6], which can be used to optimise the power consumption of the transmitter node while controlling the transmit power of the sensor nodes according to the FCC regulations for UWB transmission [7].

2.3 The IEEE 802.15.4a Standard

The IEEE 802.15.4a standard [8] is currently the most discussed and adopted standard for UWB applications in the literature. The IEEE 802.15.4a standard has been the inspiration for many UWB based MAC implementations found in the literature.

The main application of IEEE 802.15.4a is for low data rate UWB applications and ranging applications. Similar to the IEEE 802.15.6 standard, the IEEE

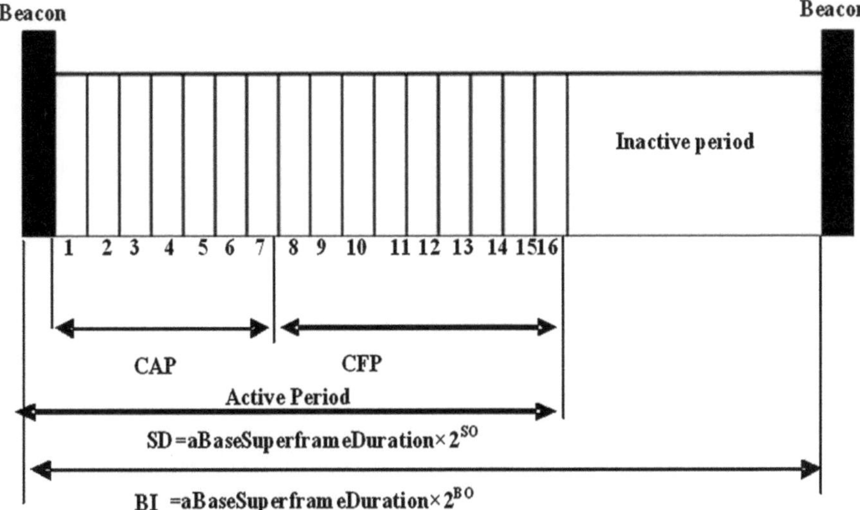

Fig. 2.2 The IEEE 802.15.4a standard super frame structure

802.15.4a standard also uses a beacon enabled super frame structure for UWB PHY layer communication. The maximum number of timeslots is limited to 16. The super frame is divided into a Contention Access Period (CAP) and a Contention Free Period (CFP). The CAP supports random access using ALOHA, while the CFP offers Guaranteed Time Slots (GTS) for high priority data traffic. The IEEE 802.15.4a standard super frame structure is shown in Fig. 2.2.

The performance of the IEEE 802.15.4a standard for WBAN applications has been intensively studied in [9, 10]. MAC layer for the IEEE 802.15.4a standard is almost identical to that of IEEE 802.15.4. The main difference is that mandatory channel access mechanism is changed to ALOHA or slotted ALOHA rather than CSMA/CA. This amendment is necessary, as it is difficult to perform CCA on the low power UWB signal.

In [9], the delay performance of the IEEE 802.15.4a standard for WBAN applications is evaluated based on two categories of physiological signals: continuous and routine signals. Physiological data such as Electrocardiography (ECG) and Electroencephalography (EEG) require continuous monitoring: hence, they are considered as continuous signals. The routine signals include body temperature and blood pressure, which are monitored periodically. The time delay is analysed based on the performance of ALOHA and slotted ALOHA channel access mechanisms on these two types of signals. The results show that the worst-case delay performance for Slotted ALOHA is better than that for the ALOHA when continuous signal data is transmitted. The performance further improves for slotted ALOHA when the number of GTS increases. The results show that when the number of GTS for slotted ALOHA is increased from 7 to 12, worst case delay drops from 75 to 25 ms. However, ALOHA has better delay performance as compared to slotted ALOHA for routine data. The results also show that the performance of slotted ALOHA degrades for routine signal as the number of GTS increases. In terms of delay, slotted ALOHA performs better for continuous signal monitoring, but not for routine signal monitoring.

Bit Error Rate (BER) analysis for on-body WBAN sensor nodes that communicate using IEEE 802.15.4a is analysed in [10]. The results show that the BER increases significantly as the number of on-body sensor nodes increases. The analysis shows that in order to maintain an acceptable BER of 10^{-3}, the maximum number of attached on-body sensor nodes has to be limited to six. The analysis is carried out based on a single user scenario where all the sensor nodes are attached to a single patient. The performance of the WBAN system will significantly degrade if there are other users in the same vicinity.

Drawbacks: The IEEE 802.15.4a standard has similar drawbacks as the IEEE 802.15.6 standard, such as the frequent use of a UWB receiver at the sensor nodes and disregarding the dynamic power control capability achievable through UWB physical layer manipulations. In addition, it does not support high data rate communication; hence restricts the extraction of the benefits provided by the UWB communications.

2.4 PSMA-Based MAC

The work presented in [11, 12] analyses the performance of an IR-UWB MAC protocol for medical data monitoring in terms throughput and power consumption. It presents a MAC protocol based on a medium access protocol called Preamble Sense Multiple Access (PSMA), where the WBAN sensor nodes sense a preamble in order to detect a busy channel or an idle channel condition. Every sensor node attaches a preamble sequence at the beginning of a data packet. The presence of this preamble code in the channel indicates a busy channel condition. The objective of using a preamble sequence is to minimize the false alarms and miss detections that can occur in traditional energy or feature based CCA methods [13]. The suggested MAC protocols in [11, 12] also uses a beacon enabled super frame structure inspired by the IEEE 802.15.4a standard. The operation of the proposed medium access method is depicted in Fig. 2.3.

The throughput and energy consumption analysis presented in [11] compares the performance of the PSMA based MAC with the slotted ALOHA based IEEE 802.15.4a standard. The comparison shows that the suggested MAC protocol performs better in terms of throughput and energy consumption for WBAN s consisting of large number of sensor nodes.

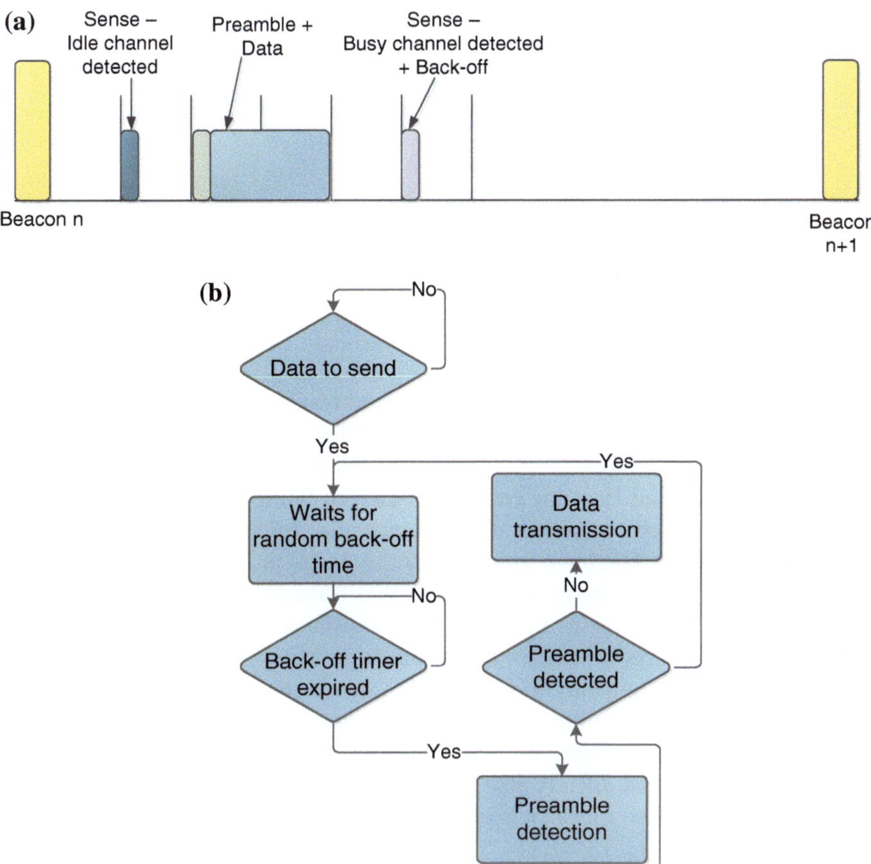

Fig. 2.3 PSMA based medium access proposed in [12], **a** data transmission using a super frame structure; **b** channel access mechanism

Drawbacks: The major drawback of this MAC protocol is that it assumes the presence of an IR-UWB based receiver at the sensor node end in order to sense the channel using PSMA mechanism. Hence, it ignores all the complexities that involve in using an IR-UWB receiver at WBAN sensor nodes that are mentioned above. It also does not provide a solution for the case where two or more sensor nodes perform preamble sense simultaneously, which leads to an eminent collision scenario.

2.5 MAC Protocol Based on Exclusion Regions

A MAC protocol developed based on transmit and receive antenna patterns and the antenna directionality is proposed in [14]. An Exclusion Region (ER) is defined as an area surrounding a receiver, such that the transmitter sensor nodes within an ER

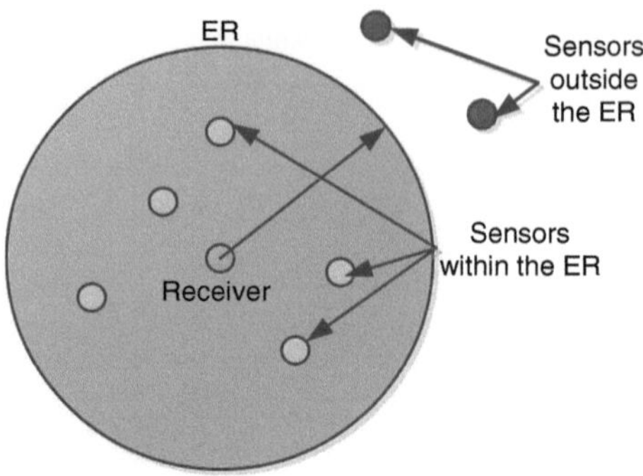

Fig. 2.4 ER based UWB communication

cause interference to each other. However, the transmitter sensor nodes that are not located inside an ER do not cause interference at the targeted receiver. In this MAC protocol, the data communication of sensor nodes within the same ER is resolved temporally using Time Hopping codes (TH-codes), while the sensor nodes in different ERs are allowed to transmit data concurrently. All the sensor nodes transmit data asynchronously. The main objective of this MAC protocol is to minimize the interference that can occur in a multiple UWB transmission environment, while optimizing the throughput using concurrent transmissions in mutually exclusive ERs. Figure 2.4 depicts the sensor communication using the ERs.

Drawbacks: Although this MAC protocol addresses the issue of interference mitigation in UWB multiple access, it does not investigate the efficiency of important factors such as pulse synchronization and multiple access for sensor nodes within the same ER. It also assumes that a sensor node can determine whether it is within the range of a certain ER by accurate ranging capabilities.

2.6 UWB^2

The Uncoordinated Wireless Baseborn Access for UWB Networks (UWB^2) protocol [15, 16] utilizes orthogonal time hopping codes in order to achieve multiple access in a shared medium. In this protocol, each node is identified using a unique TH-code, which is generated using the method provided in [17]. A common TH-code is used in order to communicate control messages and sensor initialization.

At initialization, a sensor node sends a Link Establishment (LE) frame shown in Fig. 2.5a, using the common TH-code. In this LE frame, the sensor node proposes a TH-code to be used for communication between the sensor and the coordinator. The coordinator node then replies with a Link Control (LC) message and listens to the TH-code allocated for the sensor node. The sensor initialization is followed by the data communication using the suggested TH-code and the data frame format shown in Fig. 2.5b. The UWB^2 MAC protocol supports both acknowledged and un-acknowledged data communication. The main advantage of this MAC

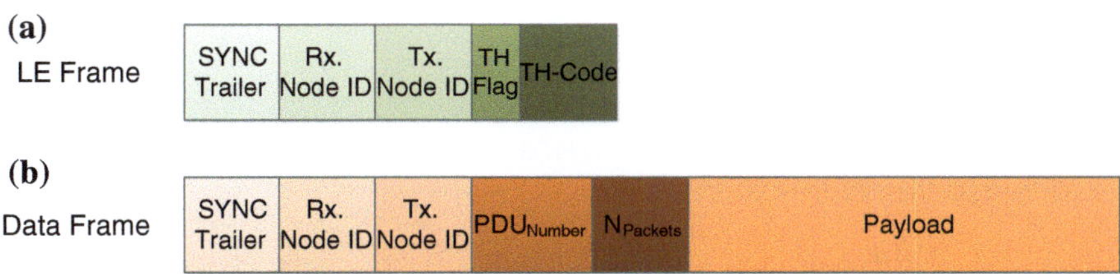

Fig. 2.5 **a** LE frame format used for sensor initialisation. **b** Data frame format

protocol is that, it has avoided the requirement for CCA by using orthogonal TH-codes. Although this MAC protocol assumes the use of a UWB receiver at the sensor node end in order to receive LC messages from the coordinator, a considerable energy saving can be achieved by avoiding the CCA. Reduced energy consumption makes it more suitable for WBAN applications.

Drawbacks: This MAC protocol does not provide a method to re-initialize the data transmission in the case of a lost LC frame. In the case of a lost LC frame, the data transmission from the sensor nodes can be inhibited permanently. In addition, collisions can occur while using the common TH-code for control messages. The MAC protocol does not suggest a method to avoid or minimize such collisions.

2.7 U-MAC

The U-MAC protocol described in [18] suggests the use of an adaptable pro-active approach for a UWB MAC design instead of a re-active approach. It is adaptable and pro-active in the sense that it suggests the dynamic allocation of transmit power and data rate at the UWB sensor nodes using *hello* messages that are used by the sensor nodes in order to advertise their local state. These messages are sent at a fixed power level, which is known to all the sensor nodes. At the reception of a *hello* message, a sensor node can determine the ranging information of the neighboring sensor nodes. This information can be used to dynamically adjust the transmit power levels of the senor nodes. This MAC protocol suggests a more sensor centric network organization approach compared to the coordinator centric approach used in other UWB based MAC protocols. This MAC protocol also supports a prioritized delivery mechanism depending on the QoS requirement of the sensor data. Similar to the UWB^2 protocol, U-MAC also uses unique TH-codes in order to provide multiple access to the shared medium, while control messages are sent using a common TH-code. Figure 2.6 demonstrates the sensor initialization procedure suggested in the MAC protocol.

On the reception of a Ready To Send (RTS) message, the neighboring sensor nodes will determine whether a new sensor node is transmitting at an admissible data rate and transmit power criteria, which are determined by the interference level and Signal to Noise Ratio (SNR) at the neighboring node. A Not Clear To

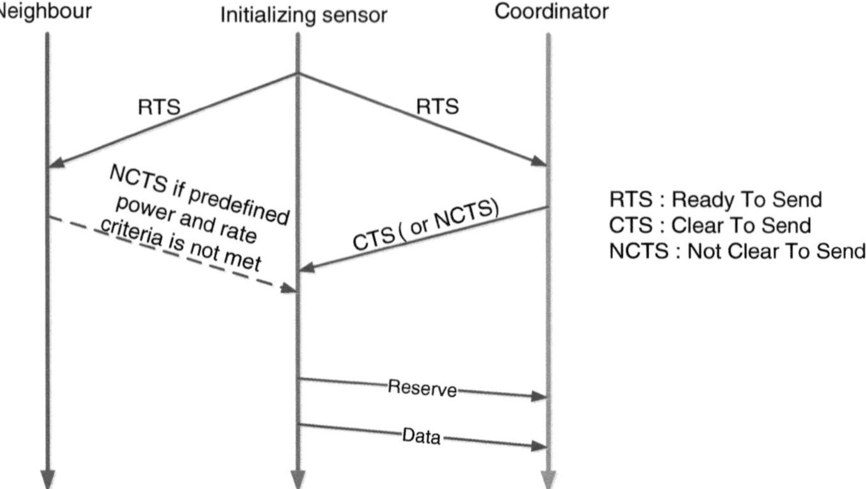

Fig. 2.6 Sensor initialization in U-MAC

Send (NCTS) message will be sent if a neighboring sensor node or a coordinator node disagrees with the parameters of the new sensor. The reception of a NCTS means that the new sensor node has to reduce it's transmit power or the data rate. If the new sensor parameters are admissible, the coordinator node will reply with a Clear To Send (CTS) message while the neighboring sensor nodes refrain from sending any messages. The data transmission occurs after the initialization. The link parameters can be dynamically adjusted during the data transmission using the *hello* messages according to the requirement of the sensor nodes.

Drawbacks: While this MAC protocol allows more dynamic usage of the UWB channel resources, it allocates significant processing load to the sensor nodes. In the context of WBANs, it is advisable to minimize the processing at the sensor node end in order to reduce power consumption. Similar to the UWB^2 MAC protocol, the U-MAC uses a UWB receiver at the sensor node end in order to receive *hello* messages and other control messages, which leads into increased power consumption and complex hardware implementation.

2.8 DCC-MAC

The DCC-MAC presented in [19, 20] uses Dynamic Channel Coding (DCC) technique in order to mitigate the multiple access interference. This MAC protocol assumes that all the sensor nodes transmit at maximum allowable transmit power in contrast to the power control mechanisms used in Sects. 2.3 and 2.6. A cross layer technique is suggested in this MAC protocol in order to mitigate the multiple access interference at the PHY layer level. The received UWB pulse amplitude is compared against a pre-defined threshold at the coordinator end. Since all the sensor nodes transmit using a pre-defined transmit power, the expected receive power for a particular sensor node can be determined by the coordinator using UWB ranging techniques. If received pulse amplitude exceeds the threshold level, it indicates a collision at the coordinator. This concept is used in the DCC-MAC in order to identify and eliminate erroneous data at the coordinator end.

Rate Compatible Punctured Convolution (RCPC) [19] codes are used in order to achieve dynamic channel coding. The multiple access to the shared medium is achieved through TH-codes as in the case of UWB^2 and U-MAC. The TH-codes are generated locally at the sensor node using a random number generator.

Drawbacks: This MAC protocol has the same drawbacks as UWB^2 and U-MAC when it comes to the use of a UWB receiver at the sensor node end. Additionally, it tries to mitigate the interference at the expense of physical layer complexity. In addition, an extensive amount of processing is allocated to the sensor nodes, which leads to an increased power consumption. It also assumes that the sensor nodes always transmit at the maximum allowable transmit power. Although this has some advantages when it comes to interference mitigation and optimizing the throughput [21], a power controlling approach might be well suited for power stringent WBAN applications of UWB. It also assumes the presence of resynchronization per every data packet, which results in increased overhead. Instead, synchronization per session is recommended for WBAN applications.

2.9   Multiband MAC for IR-UWB

Multiple access through allocation of a unique frequency band per each sensor-coordinator data communication link is suggested in [22]. A common control channel, which is assigned with a unique frequency band, is used for sensor initialization and control message transfer in this MAC protocol. Both control and data communication bands are allocated with a 500 MHz bandwidth. TH-codes are used in the common control channel in order to share it with multiple users. The main advantage of this MAC protocol is that it can be used for concurrent data transmissions from multiple numbers of sensor nodes, because of the use of different frequency bands. This assists in reducing the probability of collision, hence increases the throughput and results in low latencies, which are ideal properties for high data rate WBAN applications.

A super frame structure is used for data and control message transfer. A super frame is divided into 15 sequence frames. Each sequence is used for data transmission in each band. An *availability frame* is used between two super frames in order to indicate the availability of a particular band for data transmissions. If a sensor node intends to continue data transmission in a particular band, it has to send consecutive UWB pulses in the relevant slot allocated to indicate the occupancy of that frequency band. By sensing those UWB pulses within the corresponding time slots of the *availability frame*, other sensor nodes can determine the

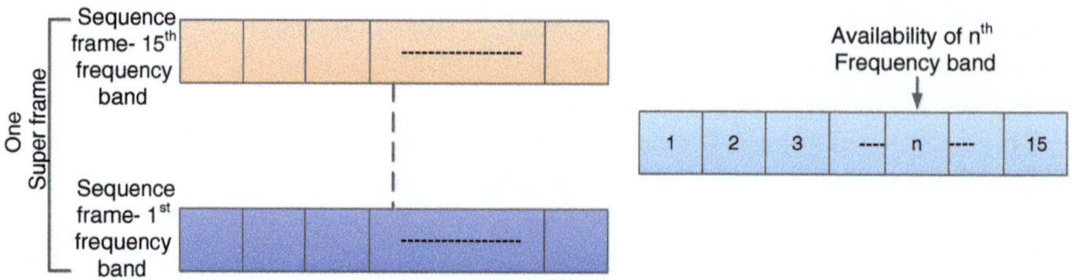

Fig. 2.7 Super frame structure used in multiband MAC

availability or occupancy of a particular band for data transmission. This super
frame structure is shown in Fig. 2.7.

Drawbacks: This MAC protocol requires the sensor nodes to operate in multiple
frequency modes in order to transmit data in different frequency bands. This
method increases the hardware complexity of the sensor nodes, which is disad-
vantageous in WBAN applications. In addition, it adds the complexity of modu-
lating the data signals into TH-codes in order to access the common control
channel. The sensor nodes have to sense the narrow UWB pulses during the
availability frame. This implies the use of a UWB receiver at the sensor node, and
energy consuming pulse-sensing procedures. Broustis et al. [22] has not specified
how the node synchronization is achieved in this MAC protocol.

2.10 Pulsers

The PULSERS project [23] uses an altered format of the IEEE 802.15.4a standard
super frame structure in order to provide high guarantee of delivery for sensor
nodes with high QoS requirements. It uses an extended CFP that facilitates GTS
for priority traffic in the IEEE 802.15.4a standard. The CAP is limited to two time
slots, where initialization messages and control messages are exchanged. When a
sensor node wants to transmit data, it requests the allocation of a GTS in the CFP
in the next super frame using the one of the time slots available in CAP. Hence,
this MAC protocol follows a Time Division Multiple Access (TDMA) based
approach in providing multiple access to the shared UWB channel.

This MAC protocol is well suited for WBAN applications with high data rate
requirements. It also proposes a peer-to-peer relay mechanism using a static
routing table, which is known to all the sensor nodes during the initialization. This
mechanism helps in decentralizing the control of the network, hence reduces the
latency. The sensor nodes can be put into inactive mode between the data transmission slots used in the MAC protocol; hence, the power consumption can be
reduced.

Drawbacks: This MAC protocol possesses all the drawbacks in the IEEE
802.15.4a standard MAC protocol when it comes to WBAN applications. The

TDMA based multiple access mechanism relies on precise synchronization in timing. However, a synchronization mechanism has not been proposed for the MAC protocol.

2.11 Transmit-only MAC

Most of the MAC protocols discussed above have limitations when it comes to UWB based WBAN applications. Many MAC protocol designs have not paid their attention towards the practical constraints that occur in hardware design. Even though IR-UWB transmitters consume low power, IR-UWB receiver needs to detect pulses with low-power level. This leads to a complex and high power consuming receiver architecture. For example, the CMOS IR-UWB transmitter discussed in [24] has a power consumption of 2 mW while the IR-UWB receivers consumes up to 32 mW of power [25]. Addition of an IR-UWB receiver in the sensor node will increase its power consumption as well as the design complexity. Implantable or wearable sensor nodes are battery powered. Hence, power consumption in sensor nodes is a critical factor that determines the efficiency of a MAC protocol. The transmit-only MAC protocol suggested in [5, 26] enables the use of a transmit-only hardware design at the sensor node end.

The suggested transmit-only MAC protocol is of asynchronous nature; hence, it faces several challenges when it comes to collision avoidance and synchronization at the receiver end. It has been designed with following characteristics in order to overcome the challenges;

- Data packets are transmitted at a much higher data rate than the required data rate so that it is possible to get an optimum sleep time for sensor nodes while it waits for the next set of data.
- Each sensor transmits at a pre allocated unique transmission slot in order to minimise the occurrence of collisions.
- A unique pulse rate is assigned for each WBAN in the same region.
- Sensor nodes transmit without prior knowledge of the channel condition.
- There is no feedback in the network.

The frame structure for this WBAN system is shown in Fig. 2.8.

When a sensor node is first connected to the network, synchronizing frame structure is used in order to assist the self-synchronization at the gateway node. A guard interval follows immediately after the initial synchronization process to allow the receiver to prepare for the reception of information in the Physical Header (PHR). The PHR contains information on the chirp rate, symbol rate, and the timing of the next transmission window. After establishing initial communication with the gateway node, the data frame will then be used in the successive transmissions. The data frame has a short preamble, which helps the receiver achieve fine synchronization followed by a guard interval to prepare the receiver

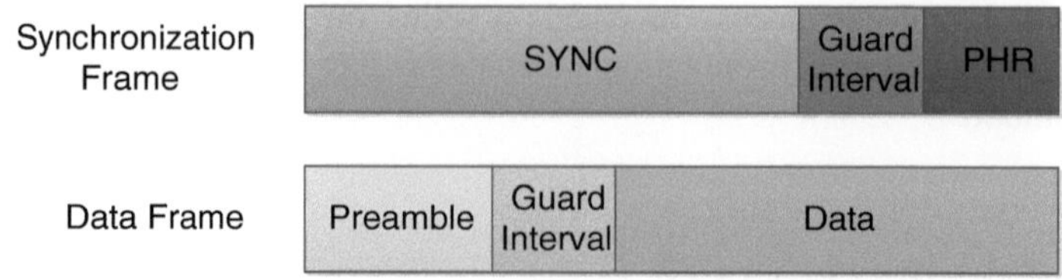

Fig. 2.8 Frame structure for Transmit-only MAC protocol for WBAN

for data reception. The data frame overhead is kept to a minimum in order to keep the transmission period short and thus reducing the chances of collision.

Drawbacks: Although the transmit-only MAC protocol addresses the problem of high power consumption, which arises due to the use of UWB receiver at the WBAN sensor node, it has several drawbacks.

- When the network traffic increases, the number of collisions, which occur due to asynchronous transmission of pulses, adversely affect the data delivery capability in the network.
- There is no feedback path to dynamically adjust the transmit power in accordance with the changing channel conditions.
- Rescheduling of the network requires manual intervention with the sensor nodes.

This MAC protocol can be further improved by the use of a narrow band receiver in order to eliminate the issues regarding the network reconfigurations and network expansion while achieving low power consumption in the sensor nodes. Such a MAC protocol is suggested in [27]. The MAC protocol described in [27] uses a narrow band receiver at the sensor node to receive feedback on properties, such as receive BER. This MAC protocol will be discussed further in Chap. 3.

2.12 Comparison of UWB-Based MAC Protocols for WBAN Applications

The MAC protocols discussed above have advantages in different areas when they are used in WBAN applications. A summary of the selected MAC schemes discussed in this section is tabulated in Table 2.1 based on their performance attributes described below.

- **Energy efficiency**—Factors affecting the energy efficiency of a MAC scheme are energy wastage due to protocol overhead, idle listening, collisions, overemitting and overhearing.
- **QoS**—Quality of Service (QoS) is crucial in a WBAN system due to the sensitivity of the data collected by sensor nodes. If the QoS is poor and the data

Table 2.1 Comparison of MAC protocols

Performance attributes	IEEE 802.15.6 [4]	IEEE 802.15.4 a [8]	PSMA based MAC [11, 12]	ER based MAC [14]	UWB^2 [15, 16]	U-MAC [18]	DCC-MAC [19, 20]	Multiband MAC [22]	PULSERS [23]	Transmit-only MAC [5, 26]	UWB-Tx and NB-Rx MAC [27]
Energy efficiency	X	X	X	X	✔	✔	X	X	X	✔	✔
Qos	✔	X	X	X	X	✔	X	X	✔	X	✔
Priority traffic	✔	✔	✔	X	X	X	X	X	✔	X	✔
Scalability	✔	X	X	✔	X	✔	X	X	X	✔	✔
Latency	X	X	X	✔	X	X	X	✔	X	✔	X
Interference mitigation	X	X	✔	✔	✔	✔	✔	✔	X	X	✔
Channel access	Random – ALOHA	Random – ALOHA	Random – PSMA	TH-code with spatial reuse	TH-code	TH-code with power management	TH-code	Frequency division	Time division	Random – Rate division	Random + TDMA

reliability is low, this could lead to a wrong diagnosis and it can be life threatening.

- **Priority traffic**—In a WBAN system, the MAC should be able to support on demand traffic and provide a method for critical data to be transmitted reliably with minimum latency.
- **Scalability**—Data rates for WBAN ranges from a few kilobytes to tens of megabytes. The number of nodes in a WBAN system can vary from a single node to tens of nodes. Therefore, scalability is an important factor to be considered in a WBAN MAC scheme.
- **Latency**—WBAN contains time critical data, therefore latency is another important factor to be considered in a WBAN MAC protocol.
- **Interference mitigation**—As the WBAN nodes are mobile, the channel condition is constantly changing. The channel condition deteriorates significantly in areas densely populated with other WBAN users. The MAC scheme should be resilient to multiple network interference.
- **Channel Access**—A WBAN constitutes of both implantable and on-body nodes. When selecting a channel access scheme, type of the nodes and the physical layer characteristics should be taken into consideration in order to ensure the reliability of the system.

2.13 Conclusion

An UWB WBAN system should be considered as a combination of a MAC protocol and the UWB hardware platform. The MAC protocols for UWB systems should be designed in a way such that it enhances the advantages provided by UWB signals and overcomes the drawbacks, specially the high complexity of a receiver. MAC protocols mentioned in this chapter have not considered manipulation of the physical layer properties of the UWB systems such as number of pulses per data bit, and transmit duty cycle, which can be incorporated with the MAC algorithm in order to make the system more dynamic in terms of data rate and QoS. These studies consider UWB for both up-link and down-link communication; hence they do not consider the complexities introduced by UWB receivers. Although the transmit-only MAC protocol suggested in [5, 24] addresses the problem of high power consumption, which arises due to the use of UWB receiver at the WBAN sensor node, it has several drawbacks. When the network traffic increases, collisions that occur due to asynchronous transmission of UWB pulses adversely affect the data delivery capability of the network. There is no feedback path to dynamically adjust the transmit signal in accordance with the changing channel conditions. Rescheduling of the network requires manual intervention with the sensor nodes. It also has to occupy different receiver nodes for each patient, since different pulse repetitive frequencies are being used to identify different users.

To avoid the use of power hungry UWB receivers and to increase the reliability of data delivery, a MAC protocol that uses a narrow band feedback path in order to communicate control messages to the sensor nodes is described in Chap. 3. With the introduction of the narrowband feedback system, it is possible to achieve a more dynamic power reduction scheme that involves cross layer designs. The use of a narrow band receiver at the sensor node end leads to simplicity of circuit design by reducing the computational complexity at the sensor node end. A dual band sensor node provides the opportunity to communicate simultaneously in the up-link and down-link reducing the communication delay. By using a narrow band receiver, in combination with a suitable MAC protocol, it is possible to achieve more dynamic network configurations; hence enable the employment of higher number of sensor nodes as well as dynamic transmit power configurations to compensate for the varying channel conditions. A narrow band receiver also provides the opportunity to manipulate various physical layer properties of UWB, such as number of IR-UWB pulses sent per data bit and duty cycle of data transmission at the sensor node; hence provide a power efficient way of controlling the performance of the network.

References

1. M.R. Yuce, T.N. Dissanayake, H.C.Keong, Wideband technology for medical detection and monitoring, recent advances in biomedical engineering. ed. by G.R Naik, ISBN: 978-953-307-004-9, InTech, 2009
2. K.M.S. Thotahewa, J.-M. Redoute, M.R. Yuce, Medium access control (MAC) protocols for ultra-wideband (UWB) based wireless body area networks (WBAN), ultra-wideband and 60 GHz communications for biomedical applications (Springer, 2013) ISBN: 978-1-4614-8895-8
3. N.J. August, H.J. Lee, D.S. Ha, Enabling distributed medium access control for impulse-based ultrawideband radios. IEEE Trans. Veh. Technol. **56**, 1064–1075 (2007)
4. http://www.ieee802.org/15/pub/TG6.html (2014)
5. H.C. Keong, M.R. Yuce, Analysis of a multi-access scheme and asynchronous transmit-only UWB for wireless body area networks. In: *31st Annual International Conference of the IEEE Engineering in Medicine and Biology Society (EMBC'09)*, pp. 6906–6909 (2009)
6. R.J. Fontana, E.A. Richley, Observations on low data rate, short pulse UWB systems. In: *IEEE International Conference on Ultra-Wideband*, pp. 334–338 (2007)
7. FCC 02-48 (First report and order) (2002)
8. IEEE-802.15.4a-2007. Part 15.4: wireless medium access control (MAC) and physical layer (PHY) specifications for low-rate wireless personal area Networks (LR-WPANs): amendment to add alternate PHY. Standard, IEEE (2014)
9. K. Takizawa, L. Huan-Bang, K. Hamaguchi, R. Kohno, wireless patient monitoring using IEEE 802.15.4a WPAN. In: *IEEE International Conference on Ultra-Wideband*, pp. 235–240 (2007)
10. D. Domenicali, M.G. Di Benedetto, Performance analysis for a body area network composed of IEEE 802.15.4a devices. In: *4th Workshop on Positioning, Navigation and Communication*, pp. 273–276 (2007)

11. L. Kynsijarvi, L. Goratti, R. Tesi, J. Iinatti, M. Hamalainen, Design and performance of contention based MAC protocols in WBAN for medical ICT using IR-UWB. In :*IEEE 21st International Symposium on Personal, Indoor and Mobile Radio Communications Workshops*, pp.107–111, 26–30 Sept 2010
12. J. Haapola, A. Rabbachin, L. Goratti, C. Pomalaza-Raez, I. Oppermann, Effect of impulse radio-ultrawideband based on energy collection on MAC protocol performance. IEEE Trans. Veh. Technol. **58**, 4491–4506 (2009)
13. B. Zhen, H.-B. Li, S. Hara, R. Kohno, "Clear channel assessment in integrated medical environments. EURASIP J. Wireless Commun. Netw. **8**(3), 1–8 (2008)
14. L.X. Cai, X. Shen, J. Mark, Efficient MAC protocol for ultra-wideband networks. IEEE Commun. Mag. **47**(6), 179–185 (2009)
15. M.-G.D. Benedetto, L.D. Nardis, G. Giancola, D. Domenicali, The aloha access (UWB)^2 protocol revisited for IEEE 802.15.4a. ST J. Res **4**(1), 131–141 (2006)
16. M.-G.D. Benedetto, L.D. Nardis, M. Junk, G. Giancola, (UWB)^2: uncoordinated, wireless, baseborn medium access for UWB communication networks. Mob. Netw. Appl. **10**(5), 663–674 (2005)
17. R. Merz, J. Widmer, J.-Y.L. Boudec, B. Radunovi'c, A joint PHY/MAC architecture for low-radiated power TH-UWB wireless ad hoc networks. Wireless Commun. Mob Comput. J. **5**(5), 567–580 (2005)
18. R. Jurdak, P. Baldi, C.V. Lopes, U-MAC: a proactive and adaptive UWB medium access control protocol. Wireless Commun. Mob Comput. J. **5**(5), 551–566 (2005)
19. J.Y.L. Boudec, R. Merz, B. Radunovic, J. Widmer, DCC-MAC: a decentralized MAC protocol for 802.15.4a-like UWB mobile ad-hoc networks based on dynamic channel coding. In: *1st International Conference on Broadband Networks*, pp. 396–405, Oct 2004
20. M. Iacobucci, M.D. Benedetto, Computer method for pseudorandom codes generation. National Italian Patent RM2001A000592, Sept 2001
21. B. Radunovic, J.Y.L. Boudec, Optimal power control, scheduling, and routing in UWB networks. IEEE J. Sel. Areas Commun. **22**(7), 1252–1270 (2004)
22. I. Broustis, S.V. Krishnamurthy, M. Faloutsos, M. Molle, J.R. Foerster, Multiband media access control in impulse-based UWB Ad Hoc networks. IEEE Trans. Mob. Comput. **6**(4), 351–366 (2007)
23. I. Bucaille, A. Tonnerre, L. Ouvry, B. Denis, MAC layer design for UWB LDR systems: PULSERS proposal. In: *4th Workshop in Positioning, Navigation and Communication*, pp. 277–283, March 2007
24. J. Ryckaert, C. Desset, A. Fort, M. Badaroglu, V. De Heyn, P. Wambacq, G. Van der Plas, S. Donnay, B. Van Poucke, B. Gyselinckx, Ultra-wide-band transmitter for low-power wireless body area networks: design and evaluation. IEEE Trans. Circuits Syst. **52**, 2515–2525 (2005)
25. G. Yuan, Z. Yuanjin, H. Chun-Huat, Low-power CMOS RF front-end for non-coherent IR-UWB receiver. In: *European Solid-State Circuits Conference*, pp. 386–389 (2008)
26. H.C. Keong, K.M.S. Thotahewa, M.R. Yuce, Transmit-only ultra wide band body sensors and collision analysis. IEEE Sens. J. **13**(5), 1949–1958 (2013)
27. K. Thotahewa, J. Khan, M. Yuce, Power efficient ultra wide band based wireless body area networks with narrowband feedback path. IEEE Trans. Mobile Comput. **PP**, 1–1 (2013) (in pre-print version)

Chapter 3
Design and Simulation of a MAC Protocol for WBAN Communication Scenarios

Abstract A Medium Access Control (MAC) protocol acts as the core of a WBAN communication system. It determines important factors that affect the efficiency of a WBAN communication system, such as throughput capability, power consumption and latency. Ultra-wideband (UWB) is a suitable wireless technology for the use in WBAN applications due to its inherent properties such as high data rate capability, low power consumption and small form factor. Although UWB transmitters are designed based on simple techniques, UWB receivers require complex hardware and consume comparatively higher power. In order to achieve reliable low power two-way communication, a sensor node can be constructed using a UWB transmitter and a narrow band receiver. This chapter presents design and simulation of a MAC protocol based on a dual-band physical layer technology. Co-simulation models based on MATLAB and OPNET have been developed to analyses the performance of the MAC protocol. The performance of the MAC protocol is analyzed for a realistic scenario where both implantable and wearable sensor nodes are involved in the data transmission. Priority based packet transmission techniques have been used in the MAC protocol to serve different sensors according to their Quality-of-Service (QoS) requirements. Analysis is done with regard to important network parameters, such as packet loss ratio, packet delay, percentage throughput, and power consumption.

Keywords MAC · UWB · Narrowband · WBAN · BER · QoS · Energy consumption · Throughput · Packet delay · PRF · Dynamic pulses per bit

3.1 Introduction

Impulse Radio-Ultra-wideband (IR-UWB) is an attractive wireless technology for WBAN applications due to its inherent features, such as low power consuming transmitter design, low complexity hardware implementation, possibility of developing sensor nodes with small form factors and high data rate capability.

K. M. S. Thotahewa et al., *Ultra Wideband Wireless Body Area Networks*, 37
DOI: 10.1007/978-3-319-05287-8_3,
© Springer International Publishing Switzerland 2014

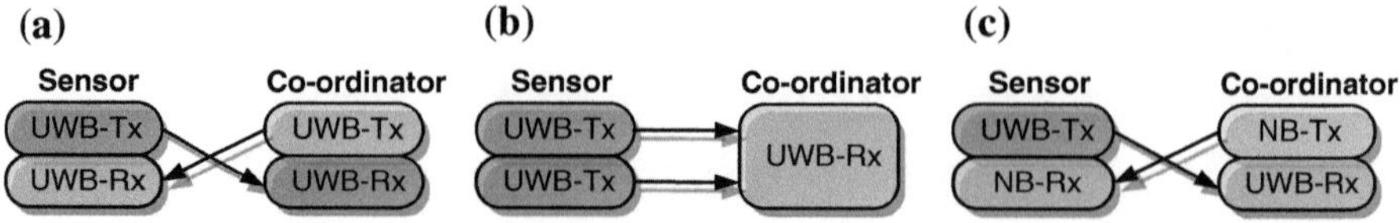

Fig. 3.1 Communication techniques for UWB based WBAN **a** sensor nodes using UWB for both transmitter and receiver **b** transmit-only method **c** sensor nodes using UWB to transmit data and narrowband to receive control messages

IR-UWB receivers are generally complex in design and consume large amount of power compared to IR-UWB transmitters. This poses a challenge to use IR-UWB technology in low-power WBAN devices. It is possible to investigate alternative approaches that lead to incorporating advantages provided by IR-UWB transmitters, while avoiding the disadvantages of using IR-UWB receivers in wearable and implantable hardware platforms [1, 2].

Figure 3.1 shows three communication protocols that can be used for an IR-UWB based WBAN. Figure 3.1a shows a standard UWB system that requires the use of a UWB transmitter and a receiver in the sensor node. Figure 3.1b is based on the UWB transmit-only technique that does not use a receiver in the sensor nodes [3, 4]. In this system, each individual sensor transmits periodically without prior knowledge of other users and the channel condition. This MAC protocol addresses the problem of high power consumption that arises due to the use of UWB receiver at the WBAN sensor node. However, it suffers from low scalability of the network, degraded performance under multiple user environments and requirement of using individual receivers for individual sensor nodes.

A very efficient technique for a UWB-WBAN network is to use a narrow band receive link instead of using UWB receiver in the sensor node side (Fig. 3.1c) [1, 5]. With the introduction of the narrowband feedback system, it is possible to achieve a more dynamic power reduction schemes that involve cross layer design. The typical current consumption of a UWB receiver is around 16 mA [2],[1] but narrowband receivers can operate at a current as low as 3.1 mA [6]; hence this can reduce the power consumption of the WBAN sensor node significantly. Using a feedback path will also reduce the computational complexity at the sensor node end. In a transmit-only system, the position of the receiver is fixed and it does not allow for reconfiguration for changing channel conditions. By using a narrow band receiver, the gateway node can use the narrowband feedback to reconfigure the system to adapt to changing channel conditions without any user intervention. It is also important to note that the feedback path does not require high data rate since it will be mostly used for sending acknowledgement and control messages. A simple narrowband receiver does not consume much of additional design space. It also

---

[1] UWB receivers consume more power than narrow-band receivers as the transmission of UWB signal has low power levels as well as the higher operation frequency.

consumes very small power since it is only powered on when required (for example, sleep mode operation in a periodic data transmission).

Compared to the transmit-only method a UWB WBAN system with narrowband feedback improves the network and reduces collisions. It also helps to optimize the power consumption of the sensor node, introducing additional power savings. In a system where both transmitter and the receiver use UWB, a turnaround time should be used to switch from transmit state to receive state. In other words, transmitter and receiver cannot operate at the same time due to the interference. Since we are using a narrow band receiver, it is possible to operate both transmitter and receiver simultaneously; hence reducing the packet delay. Also, independent downstream/upstream communication enables a much simpler MAC design.

The MAC protocol presented in this chapter is unique in the sense that it is developed to enhance the performance of a WBAN using the high data rate offered by the UWB transmission while using a narrowband feedback path to avoid the complexities given by a UWB receiver. In this MAC protocol, the priority of data is taken into consideration and a guaranteed delivery mechanism is utilised to transfer data with high priority. Different topologies are simulated in order to investigate various performance indicators of the network design such as throughput, power consumption and delay.

3.2 Simulation Models

Simulations presented in this chapter are conducted in a co-simulation approach using Matlab [7] and Opnet Modeler [8], which are commercially available simulation softwares. Physical layer simulations are done in Matlab. Matlab is linked to Opnet Modeler using "MX interface" provided in Matlab. Opnet Modeler runs in interactive co-simulation with Matlab for networking performance analysis and it calls Matlab for physical layer performance. During a simulation, Opnet executes as the master simulator, and invokes Matlab engine server to execute the UWB transmitter developed in Simulink [7]. Opnet then takes back the control of the simulation and executes networking functions. At the receiver stage, Opnet again calls Matlab to execute UWB pulse receiver block. Output data bits of the receiver stage are then used to generate the received data packets.

3.2.1 IR-UWB Pulse Generation

IR-UWB transmit pulse generation is achieved using Matlab, which is then used in co-simulation with Opnet Modeler. This pulse generation technique is shown in Fig. 3.2. An IR-UWB signal with a bandwidth of 1 GHz centered at 4 GHz is considered for the simulations. The pulse repetitive frequency (PRF), pulse width

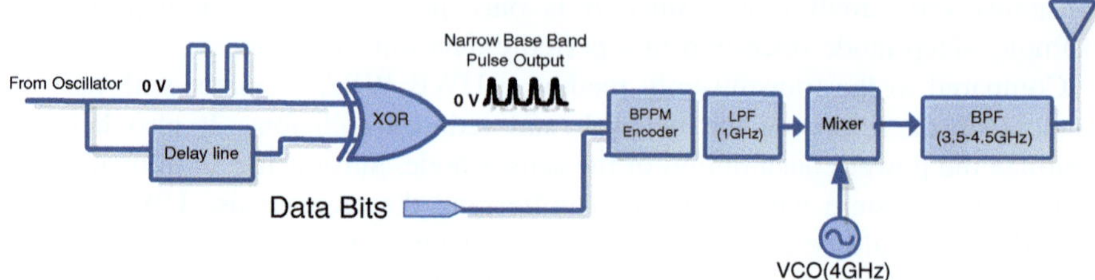

Fig. 3.2 IR-UWB pulse generation technique

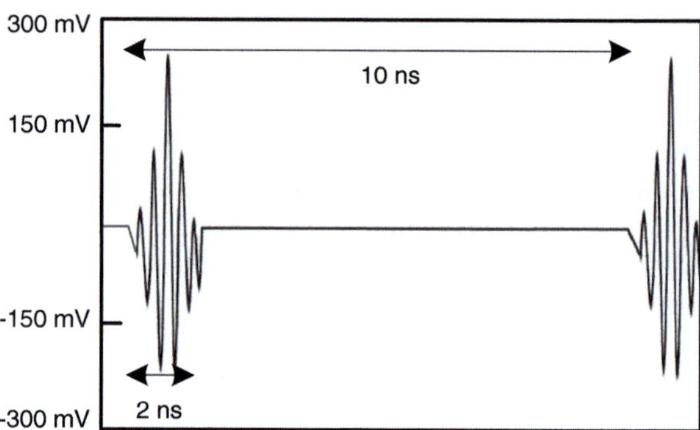

Fig. 3.3 IR-UWB pulse stream generated by the simulated pulse generator

and rise time of the UWB pulses affect the output transmit spectrum [9, 10]. Pulse properties are chosen considering the information given in [9]. For the simulations described in this chapter, a PRF of 100 MHz, a pulse width of 2 ns and a rise time of 100 ps is chosen. Figure 3.3 depicts an example IR-UWB pulse stream generated by the simulated pulse generator model. The data packets generated in the Opnet environment is combined with IR-UWB pulses and then transmitted over the propagation channel described in the following subsection.

3.2.2 Propagation Channel Model

Figure 3.4 depicts different types of nodes simulated in this chapter. Both implanted and wearable sensor nodes are considered during the simulations. Coordinator node and router nodes are placed outside the body. Three types of propagation channel models are developed in order to simulate different propagation characteristics that exist in the simulation environment. These propagation channels are depicted in Fig. 3.5.

Propagation channel for the transmission of in-body signals (propagation channel 1) is developed using information presented in [11]. Two implanted sensor nodes at 5 and 80 mm implant depths are considered for the simulations. The path loss at a distance d in propagation channel 1 ($P_{dB}(d)$) can be calculated as;

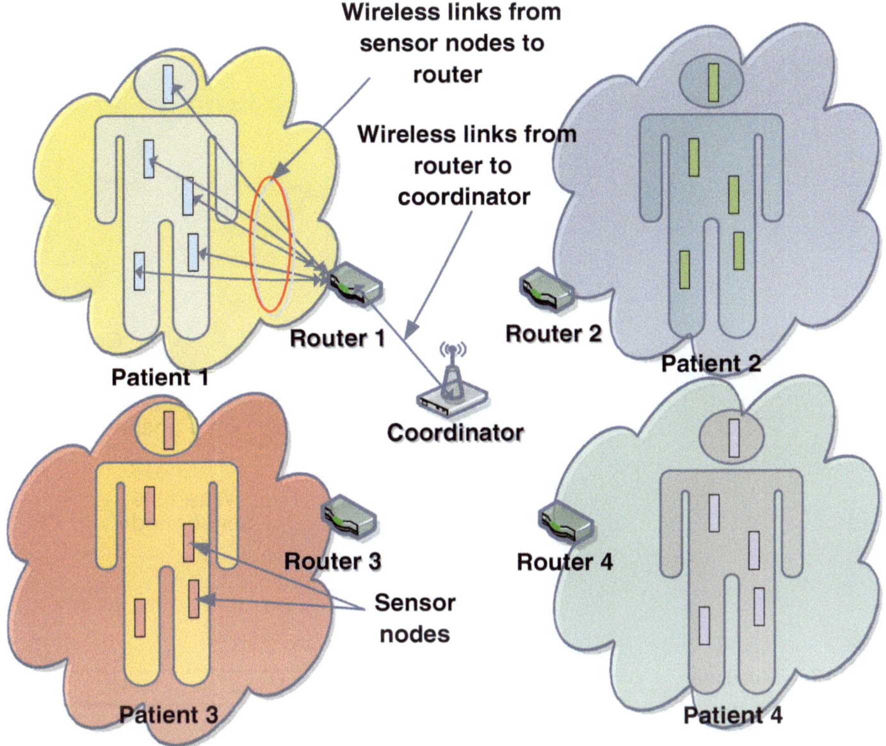

Fig. 3.4 Topology of WBAN for a multi-human monitoring environment

$$P_{dB}(d) = P_{0,dB} + a\left(\frac{d}{d_0}\right)^n + N\big(\mu(d), \sigma^2(d)\big) \tag{3.1}$$

where d is the depth from the skin in millimeters, d_0 is the reference distance (5 mm), $P_{0,dB}$ is the path loss at reference distance in dB, a is the fitting constant, n is the path loss exponent and $N(\mu(d), \sigma^2(d))$ is a normally distributed random variable with a mean of μ and a standard deviation of σ. Parameters in Table 3.1 are used during the simulations [11].

An indoor propagation channel model for UWB communication based on the modified Saleh-Valenzuela model is developed for propagation channels 2 and 3 in Fig. 3.5. It consists of a discreet impulse response given by (3.2) [12]. Considering an average communication distance of 2 m, statistical channel measurements for CM1 channel model [13] is taken as the reference.

$$h_i(t) = X_i \sum_{p=0}^{K} \sum_{q=0}^{L} a_{p,q}^i \delta\big(t - T_p^i - \tau_{p,q}^i\big) \tag{3.2}$$

Fig. 3.5 Propagation channels implemented in the simulations

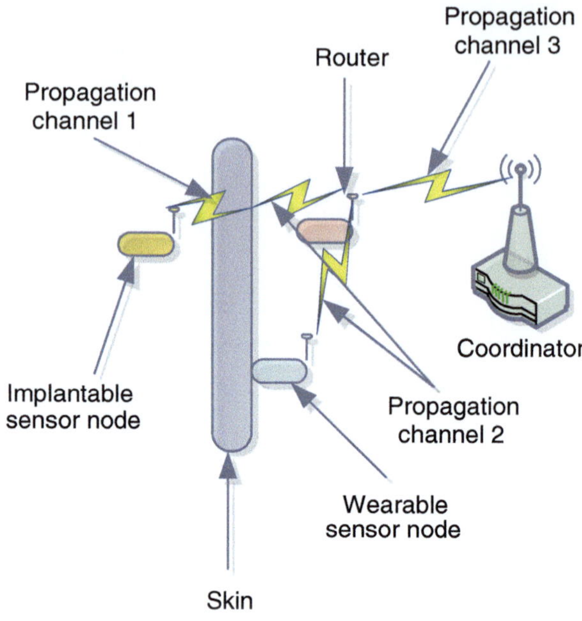

Table 3.1 Simulation parameters for in body propagation channel

Parameter	Value
$P_{0,dB}$	6.3 dB
a	11.6
n	0.5
d	5 mm/80 mm
μ	d = 5 mm:2.7, d = 80 mm:8.2
σ	d = 5 mm:5, d = 80 mm:6.6

where X_i represents lognormal shadowing, $a^i_{p,q}$ are the multipath gain coefficients, T^i_p represents delay of the pth IR-UWB pulse, $\tau^i_{p,q}$ is the delay of the qth multipath relative to pth pulse arrival time and 'i' refers to the ith realization of the channel.

The average path loss (L) of IR-UWB signals at a distance of d for this model is given by (3.3) [13]:

$$L1 = 20\log\left(\frac{4\pi f_c}{c}\right), \ L2 = 20\log(d) \text{ and } L = L_1 + L_2 \tag{3.3}$$

where $f_c = \sqrt{f_{min} * f_{max}}$ is the geometric centre frequency of the waveform, f_{min} and f_{max} are the -10 dB edges of the waveform spectrum, c is the speed of light, L_1 is the path loss at 1 m distance and d is the distance relative to 1 m reference point. When the simulations are conducted for the scenario where implanted sensor nodes directly communicate with the coordinator or router node placed

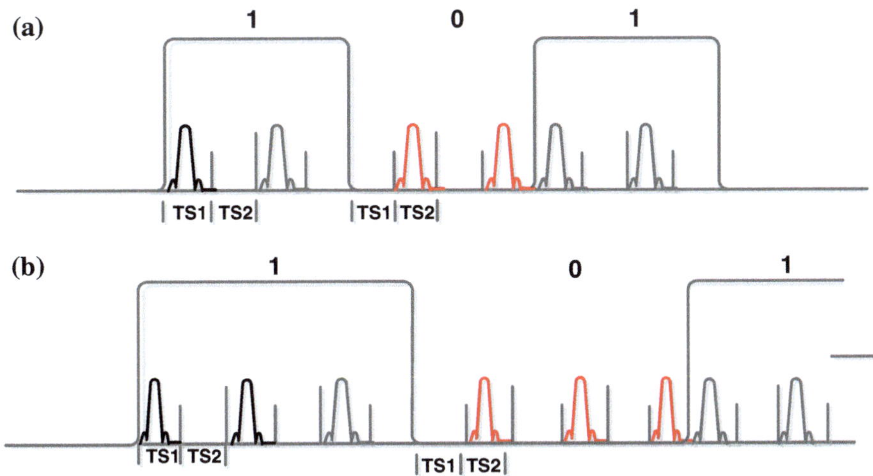

Fig. 3.6 Pulse train for '1' '0' '1' bit pattern using **a** two PPB and **b** three PPB in BPPM

outside the body, in-body propagation model is used for the distance up to the surface of the skin, and indoor model is used for rest of the distance.

Amplitude Shift Keying (ASK) scheme is used for the narrow band communication, which operates based on the 433 MHz ISM band. The power level for the narrowband signal is kept at -25 dBm, which is a reasonable value for operation with less interference. Ricean fading channel for indoor propagation [14] is used to simulate the propagation in the narrowband channel. The narrow band signal for in-body communication is assumed to follow the free space channel model.

3.3 Cross Layer Design

The MAC protocol described in this chapter incorporates unique physical layer properties of UWB transmission in its design. Hence, it forms a cross layer architecture. A simple Binary Pulse Position Modulation (BPPM) technique is used as the modulation scheme for the UWB transmission. This eliminates the complexities introduced by the use of complex modulation schemes for low power WBAN applications. The sensor nodes in the simulations use two mechanisms to ensure that the transmit power is managed effectively. The first mechanism is to use a gated pulse transmission scheme, where a sensor node transmits the UWB data for a given time period and go into low power mode till the next transmission slot. A dynamically varying multiple pulses per bit (PPB) scheme is used as the second scheme in order to optimize the transmit power consumption by controlling the bit transmission time. These two mechanisms are discussed in detail under this section. Figure 3.6 depicts the use of 2 and 3 PPB schemes for sending data bits.

3.3.1 Transmission Power Regulations of the Gated UWB Pulse Transmission

According to the Federal Communications Commission (FCC) regulations a UWB signal is power limited by measured Full Bandwidth (FBW) peak power of 0 dBm (1 mW) and measured average power density of -41.25 dBm/MHz (75 nW/MHz) [15, 16]. These power measurements assume a resolution bandwidth of 1 MHz and an integration time of 1 ms for the measuring equipment.

The peak emission limit of a UWB signal depends on the resolution bandwidth of the spectrum analyzer and varies according to (3.4) [16]:

$$P_{peak} = 20 \; \log\left(\frac{B_R}{50}\right) \; \text{dBm} \tag{3.4}$$

where P_{peak} is the peak power limit and B_R is the resolution bandwidth of the spectrum analyzer. For average power measurements, a resolution bandwidth of 1 MHz and an integration time of 1 ms should be used while the resolution bandwidth can be varied between 1 and 50 MHz according to (3.4). A data packet is transmitted at much shorter time than the integration time of 1 ms as recommended by the FCC regulations. The data transmission resembles a gated system where a sensor node transmits a data packet within a very short time slot and switches off the transmitter till the next transmission slot. If P^m_{peak} is the measured peak power and P^m_{avg} is the measured average power, the maximum allowable UWB transmit power for a system with much higher PRF than the resolution bandwidth of the spectrum analyzer can be given by (3.5) [16]:

$$P_{peak} = \frac{P^m_{peak}}{\tau R} = \frac{P^m_{avg}}{\tau R} \tag{3.5}$$

where P_{peak} is the actual maximum transmit power of the UWB signal, τ is the UWB pulse width and R is the pulse repetitive frequency. This equation suggests the peak emission power limit for a continuous transmission system, but not for a gated system such as the system described in this chapter. An update to the original FCC standards is made in 2005 allowed using higher transmit power for gated UWB systems [17]. If δ represents the duty cycle of the packet transmission based on an integration time of 1 ms, it can be seen from (3.6) that the total allowable transmit power is much higher for a gated system than that of a non-gated system.

$$P_{peak} = \frac{P^m_{avg}}{\tau R \delta} \tag{3.6}$$

The UWB based WBAN sensor node design example given in this chapter is simulated with a PRF of 100 MHz, which is comparably high relative to a resolution bandwidth of 1 MHz. Hence it is considered a high PRF system. These

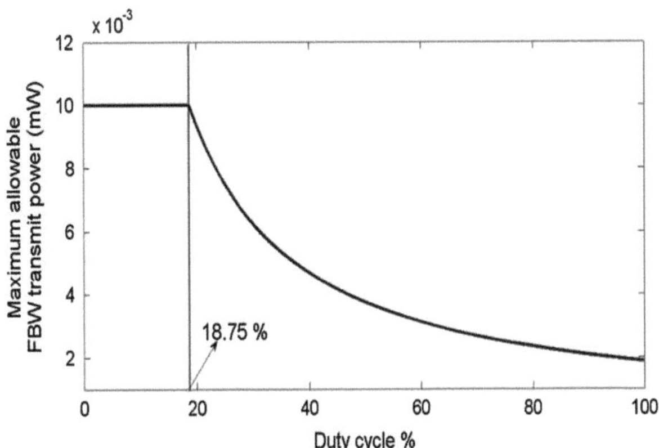

Fig. 3.7 Variation of full bandwidth peak power with duty cycle

measured power limitations can be converted to maximum allowable FBW transmit power limits using (3.7) and (3.8) [16, 18];

$$P_{peak} \leq 7.5 \times 10^{-8} \left(\frac{B_p}{R}\right)^2 \times \frac{1}{\delta} \ \text{W} \qquad (3.7)$$

$$P_{peak} \leq 0.001 \left(\frac{B_R}{50 \times 10^6}\right)^2 \times \left(\frac{B_p}{R}\right)^2 \ \text{W} \qquad (3.8)$$

where $B_p = 1/\tau$. The maximum allowable FBW transmit power is governed by smaller of the two P_{peak} values in (3.7) and (3.8).

For the simulated system, a pulse width of 2 ns is used. Hence B_p in (3.7) and (3.8) is equal to 0.5 GHz for the UWB signals used in the simulations. Figure 3.7 shows the variation of maximum allowable FBW transmit power values with the duty cycle (δ) for a sensor node that generates UWB signals with a PRF of 100 MHz and a pulse width of 2 ns. Resolution bandwidth (B_R) is taken as 1 MHz according to the FCC specifications. According to Fig. 3.7, the transmit slot of the UWB data should be kept within 187.5 μs (micro seconds) in order to transmit at maximum allowable power of 0.01 mW that complies with the FCC limitations.

3.3.2 BER Analysis of Multiple PPB Scheme

Since the power required to transmit a data bit is equal to the summation of the power of number of pulses sent to represent that data bit, a considerable power saving can be achieved if allocation of the number of PPB can be dynamically changed according to the minimum Bit Error Rate (BER) requirement at the receiver end. The timing parameters, that are used in this MAC protocol is decided using this calculation and are further described in this section. An energy-detecting

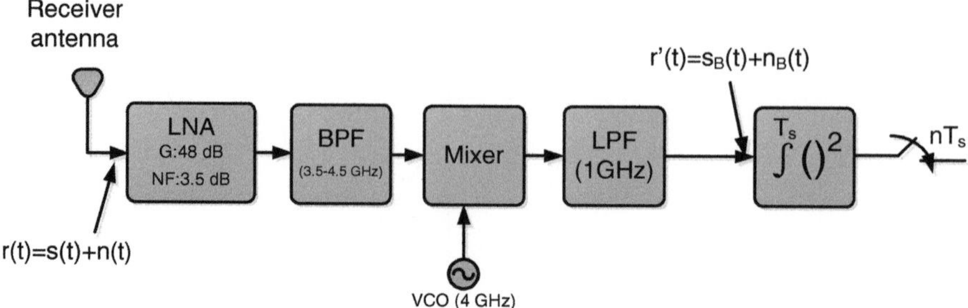

Fig. 3.8 The energy detection receiver architecture used in the simulations

receiver is used as the receiver model for the simulations (Fig. 3.8) [19]. The integration duration (T_s) for the receiver is 2 ns, which is equal to the pulse width of the UWB signal. The small integration time helps to reduce the multipath interference that might occur during UWB communication.

The bit errors in a WBAN environment mainly occur due to multipath interference and random fading of the UWB signal that originates from reflection from various surfaces and different absorption characteristics of objects, such as various body surfaces and indoor equipment. Assume that a sensor node transmits data with a sufficient transmit power for the signal to be detected by the receiver node in an ideal free space scenario without fading and multipath interference. Also, assume that two identical sets of data are transmitted using the same transmit power and same separation distance as above in a realistic WBAN environment that is susceptible to multipath interference and random fading with one data set transmitted using a higher PPB value and the other with a lower PPB value. The transmit signal with higher PPB transmission results in a lower BER than a lower PPB transmission for the same separation distance in a realistic environment with fading and multipath interference. Consider the energy detection receiver architecture shown below:

The input to the band pass filter at the UWB receiver of the parent node can be expressed as:

$$r(t) = \begin{cases} n(t) & \textit{if there is no pulse present} \\ & \textit{in a time slot} \\ s(t) + n(t) & \textit{if there is a pulse present} \\ & \textit{in a time slot} \end{cases} \tag{3.9}$$

where $r(t)$ is the input to the band pass filter, $s(t)$ is the received UWB signal and $n(t)$ is the Additive White Gaussian Noise (AWGN) with zero mean and a flat power spectral density of $N_0/2$. The received signal is then sent through a Band Pass Filter (BPF) with a 1 GHz bandwidth centered at 4 GHz. Then it is down converted into a base band signal using a mixer. A Low Pass Filter (LPF) with a bandwidth of 1 GHz is applied before the integrator. The received signal at the input to the integrator can be given by:

$$
r'(t) = \begin{cases} n_B(t) & \textit{if there is no pulse present} \\ & \textit{in a time slot} \\ s_B(t) + n_B(t) & \textit{if there is a pulse present} \\ & \textit{in a time slot} \end{cases} \tag{3.10}
$$

where $n_B(t)$ is the band-limited noise signal and $s_B(t)$ is the filtered received signal. With the assumption that the receiver node detects the presence of a pulse by comparing the signal energies of the two BPPM slots (TS1 and TS2), probability of error for single pulse detection of the receiver with BPPM modulation scheme can be derived from [20] :

$$
P_e = Q\left(\sqrt{ \frac{\left(E_p/N_0 \right)^2}{2\left(E_p/N_0 + T_s B \right)} } \right) \tag{3.11}
$$

where P_e is the probability of error, B is the signal bandwidth ($B = 1$ GHz for the receiver model used in the simulations), T_s is the integration period which is equal to the pulse width of 2 ns for the simulations, E_p is the received signal energy during the 2 ns integration period (T_s) and Q ( ) represents the Q function. It should be noted that the system described in [20] uses the detection of multiple pulses during a single integration period, whereas the system presented in this chapter detects only a single pulse within the integration period. For the system in [20], the noise-by-noise product term increases due to the detection of multiple pulses within the same integration window, significantly reducing the BER performance of the system. Due to the independent detection of individual pulses and using those individual detections to determine the presence of a bit, the noise by noise product term does not affect the system presented in this chapter. Hence, the BER equation presented in [20] reduces to (3.11) in this chapter for a single pulse detection system.

When multiple PPB is sent, it is assumed that a bit is erroneous when more than half the pulses sent per that bit are erroneous. If N pulses are sent per bit, probability that a bit being erroneous can be obtained by:

$$
P_{e_{bit}} = 1 - \sum_{i=1}^{\left\lfloor \frac{N}{2} \right\rfloor} \binom{N}{i} p^i (1-p)^{N-i} \tag{3.12}
$$

where $p = P_e$, $\binom{N}{i} = \frac{N!}{i!(N-i)!}$ and $\lfloor x \rfloor$ is the inferior integer part of x. Modulation curves showing BER for different number of PPB are obtained based on (3.12) and presented in Fig. 3.9. It should be noted that the BER is plotted against pulse E_p/N_0 in this figure. Bit energy can be obtained by the summation of pulse energies that represent the bit. The results in Fig. 3.9 show that for the same E_p/N_0, sending more number of PPB results in lower BER.

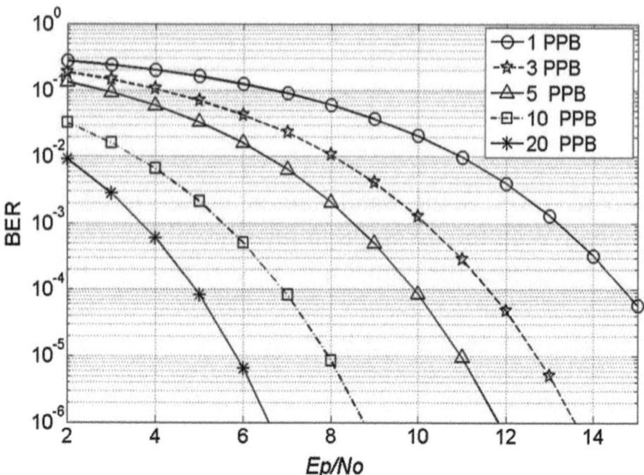

Fig. 3.9 Bit Error Rate (BER) versus pulse Ep/No (dB) curves for different number of PPB

The bit-error-rate calculation based on (3.11) does not consider the Multiple Access Inference (MAI) caused by other users and the Multi Path Interference (MPI). This interference can be modelled using a normal distribution as $\sim N(0, M)$, where M depends on received energy from interferers and multipaths [20]. Hence (3.11) can be modified into (3.13) with the consideration of MAI and MPI.

$$P_e = Q\left(\sqrt{\frac{\left(E_P/N_0\right)^2}{2\left(E_P/N_0 + T_sB\right) + M}}\right) \tag{3.13}$$

Given that the WBAN is limited to a short range of 0–2 m, and the network topology in the simulations are arranged such that the coordinator is placed at the center while the patients with the sensor nodes are placed around the coordinator preserving the Line-Of-Sight (LOS), the presence of a strong LOS component together with the multipath components is assumed in the simulations.

3.3.3 Determination of Pulses Per Bit Values by Parent Node

According to the analysis shown above, the energy consumption of a UWB transmitter is determined by two limiting factors. Firstly, the maximum allowable FBW transmit power, which depends on the duty cycle of the pulse transmission, determines the maximum limit of the energy per UWB pulse. Secondly, the number of PPB value determines the number of UWB pulses sent within the pulse transmission slot, which determines the energy consumption within the transmission slot. However, these two factors are inter-dependent. Both these factors have to be considered when determining the transmission slot duration and the duty cycle for a certain sensor node that requires a specific data rate. However, dynamically changing the FBW transmit power involves the use of a variable gain amplifier at the sensor node end in a practical scenario, while dynamically changing the PPB value can be done by varying the bit duration of the bits generated using a microcontroller of a sensor node. The latter is simpler to implement and less power consuming than the former. Hence, FBW transmit value is kept constant within the limits specified in Sect. 3.3.1 for the sensor nodes considered in the simulations. The PPB value is dynamically changed in order to optimize the power consumption of the sensor node.

In the WBAN system described in this chapter, a parent node dynamically assigns the number of PPB for a child node in order to obtain a specified optimum BER value at the receiver. A BER threshold of 10^{-4} is used in the simulation scenario for all sensor nodes, because a good throughput can be obtained with this value while keeping the power consumption at the sensor nodes low. During the data transmission, the sensor nodes insert a certain number of bytes containing a known bit patterns equally spread among the data bits. For the simulations, six bytes are chosen for continuous sensors while three bytes are chosen for periodic sensors. A parent node dynamically determines the BER for a particular sensor node using the known bit pattern, and compares it against the 10^{-4} threshold. Note that this calculated BER value includes the bit errors due to MPI, MAI as well as the noise characteristics. Sensor nodes start data transmission with the highest allowable PPB value for that particular sensor type during an allocated transmission slot for that sensor node (time slot allocation is discussed in a following section). Coordinator node requests a particular sensor node to dynamically reduce the PPB value in 1 PPB steps until a BER value of 10^{-4} or the closest possible value which is higher than the 10^{-4} threshold is achieved using the minimum PPB value possible. This procedure ensures that the sensor nodes transmit data using the minimum achievable PPB while maintaining a close to 10^{-4}. The sensor nodes resend the same data packet until an agreement is made to use a certain PPB value for future data transmissions. In the case of degradation in the BER during data transmission using the pre agreed PPB, parent node repeats the above process to increase the PPB value to improve the BER. If a certain sensor node receives a message to increase the previously assigned PPB value, it resends the previously sent data packet modulated according to the new assignment. Note that changing the PPB value is achieved in sensor nodes by varying the duration of the bit, not the PRF. Hence, the receiver node does not have to change the sampling frequency for each sensor node. It keeps track of the number of PPB assigned to each sensor node. This can be achieved in the MAC layer. As a result, a single receiver node can be utilised for all the sensor nodes. The dynamic BER compensation procedure described above is particularly useful in short range UWB communications systems where a strong LOS path is present, such as the WBAN system described in this chapter, to achieve reliable communication during dynamic channel conditions.

Table 3.2 Commonly monitored medical parameters

Medical parameter	Transmit period	Sampling rate (samples/s)	Bits per sample	Data rate
WCE	Continuous			5 Mbps
ECG	Continuous	300	12	3.6 kbps
EEG	Continuous	200	12	2.4 kbps
Heart beat	Every 1 s			100 bps
Oxygen saturation	Every 1 s			100 bps
Blood pressure	Every 1 min			12 bps
Temperature	Every 1 min			12 bps

3.3.4 Super Frame Structure

A Beacon enabled super frame structure is considered for the UWB WBAN MAC protocol. The network topology for the simulated system is developed based on a simplified version of the IEEE 802.15.4/4a [21, 22] beacon enabled star topology with modifications added to make it better suited for low power IR-UWB transmission. Beacon enabled mode provides the timeliness guarantees to the network.

Super frame structure depends on three major factors; the data rate and priority requirements of the sensor nodes, duty cycle requirement, which itself depends on the maximum power limitations and finally, the total number of active sensor nodes in the network.

A set of commonly monitored physiological parameters are shown in Table 3.2. A WBAN consists of two types of sensor nodes depending on their data transmission rate. WCE, ECG and EEG[2] are continuously transmitting sensors that require high data transmission rate and high guarantee of delivery [3]. These signals can be classified as critical parameters and the MAC protocol is designed to prioritize the delivery of such data. Sensor nodes that transmit heart rate and blood pressure are periodic sensors and do not require high data rate.

The super frame structure described in this section is divided into a Contention Access Period (CAP) and a Contention Free Period (CFP). CFP offers Guaranteed Time Slots (GTS) for the sensor nodes to transmit data. Continuously transmitting sensor nodes are thus assigned with GTS to increase the reliability of the network. Periodic sensor nodes contend for transmission during the CAP.

Data rates for the sensor nodes in the simulation are chosen in order to represent the sensor nodes that require highest data rates from each type. This means, an effective data rate of 5 Mbps is chosen for a continuous sensor node and it is assumed that the periodic sensor nodes produce 100 bits every one second. However, this 100-bit payload for a particular periodic sensor node is sent during one time slot in the CAP to increase the efficiency of the MAC protocol.

---

[2] These continuous medical signals are usually considered as crucial in hospital environments. However classification of medical signals can easily be prioritised according to the individual patient being monitored.

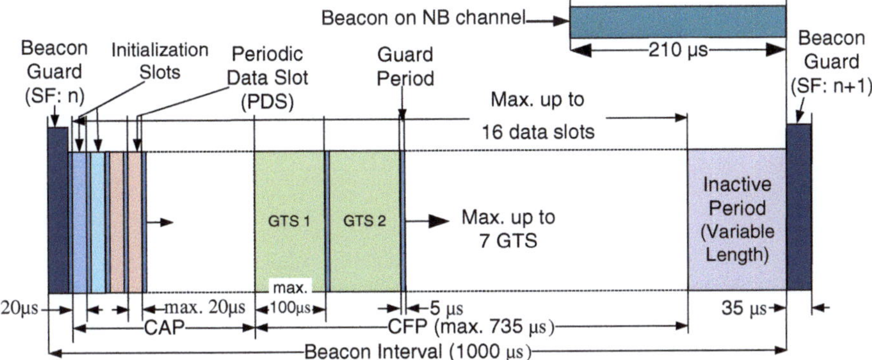

Fig. 3.10 Super frame structure

The total length of the super frame including the beacon is kept at 1 ms. The transmit slot durations for each sensor node type is decided based on the data rate requirement, peak transmit power limitation and allowed PPB value range for a particular sensor type. The duty cycle for all the sensor nodes is kept equal or below the threshold limit of 18.75 % in order to utilize the maximum power limit according to the analysis in Sect. 3.3.1.

For example, consider the case of a continuous sensor transmitting at 5 Mbps. The allowable set of PPB values is chosen to be 1 and 2 PPB for this sensor type, considering the data rate requirement, duty cycle requirement and the need to facilitate the data transfer for multiple sensor nodes within the super frame. When a continuous sensor node is transmitting at 2 PPB, which is the maximum allowable PPB value, it needs to transmit 10,000 pulses every 1 ms in order to achieve the given data rate of 5 Mbps. At a PRF of 100 MHz this can be done within a 100 μs time slot, resulting in a duty cycle of 10 %. However, if a continuous sensor node is transmitting at 1 PPB, it will transfer data in a 50 μs time slot. Similarly a maximum of 20 μs time slot duration is chosen for periodic sensor nodes assuming a PPB range of 1–20 PPB. A larger PPB value range is allocated for periodic sensor nodes in order to compensate for the possible increase in interference level that might occur during the CAP. Two initialization slots of fixed 20 μs duration are allocated at the beginning of the super frame for sensor initialization. Initialization requests are sent during these two time slots at a fixed 20 PPB value. This value is assumed to be known to all the sensor nodes. The synchronization beacons are sent using the narrow band channel in parallel with the UWB transmission in order to reduce the data rate requirement of the narrow band feedback (Fig. 3.10). Narrow band beacon duration of 0.210 ms is used in the simulations, which contains 4 bits transmitting at 19.2 kbps [6]. The CAP for each super frame starts after a fixed 35 μs beacon guard slot from the end of the beacon period. A fixed guard period of 5 μs is allocated at the end of each time slot. This super frame structure is shown in Fig. 3.10. Note that it is the maximum time slot duration that determines the maximum limit of time slots that can be

Fig. 3.11 Main algorithms used in the UWB-MAC simulation environment for **a** sensor initialization of continuous sensors **b** data delivery of continuous sensors **c** data delivery of periodic sensors

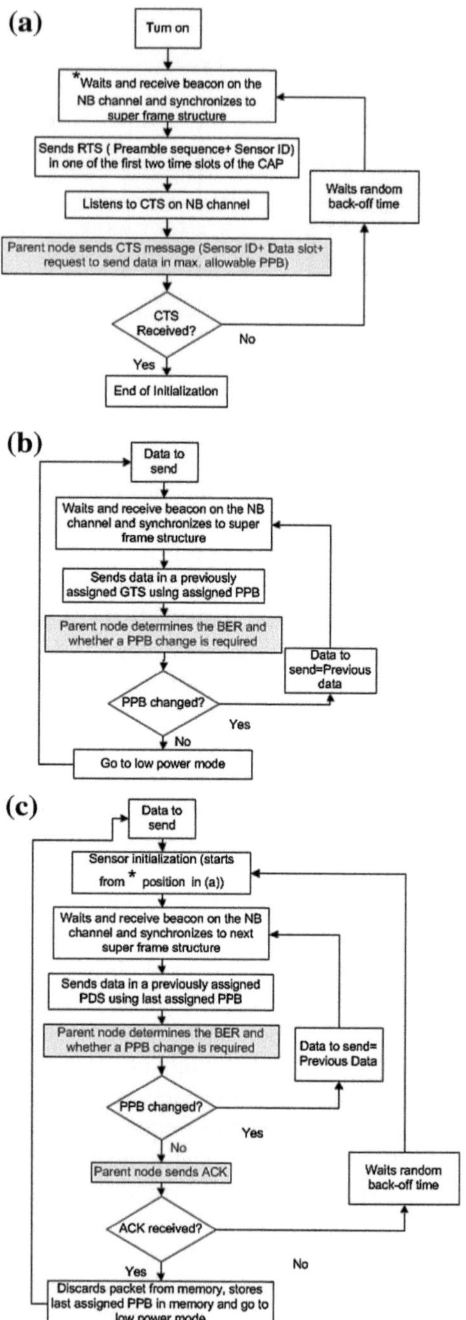

accommodated within the super frame for each sensor type. The number of timeslots allocated for each sensor type is discussed under a following section.

3.3.5 Medium Access Control Algorithm

Two different addressing levels are required in order to identify the sensor nodes used in the WBAN. One addressing level identifies the patient while the other addressing level identifies the different sensors that belong to the same patient. In the simulation model, 9-bit address space is used as the source. In this 9-bit address space, six least significant bits are used to identify the sensor while three most significant bits are used to identify the patient. Due to the use of the dual band method, it is not possible to do a carrier sensing at the sensor node end without using additional hardware. Additional hardware adds more power overhead. Hence a random access method is developed to access the medium during the contention access period. Maximum retransmissions are limited to four during sensor initialization. This value is supported by the IEEE 802.15.4 standard [21] and is identified in the simulations as a sufficient value to achieve reliable communication. A super frame supports up to seven GTS. Allocation of GTS is done by the coordinator on the request of sensor nodes. GTS slot allocation is dynamically done according to the demand so that all other remaining time slots can be used for random access. All the sensor nodes are initialized during the first two time slots of the super frame using random access. Continuously transmitting sensor nodes will request for GTS from the coordinator during the initialization. Periodic sensor nodes will transmit using random access during the CAP slot. Figure 3.11 depicts the algorithms used for sensor initialization and data transmission of continuous and periodic sensors.

During the initialization, a pre-defined PPB value (20 PPB in the simulations) is used by the sensor nodes to communicate with its parent node. This value is known to both sensor node and its parent node. A known bit pattern appended by a pre-defined sensor address and sensor type flag (continuous or periodic) is sent in the initialization request. As a response to the initialization request, parent node will send a positive or negative acknowledgement. If the request is from a continuous sensor node, parent node will permanently assign a time slot in CFP for that particular sensor node. For periodic sensors, a time slot for the next cycle of data transmission will be reserved by the coordinator node. After initialization, PPB assignment is done as discussed in the Sect. 3.3.3 and data transmission continues.

3.4 Simulation Scenarios and Performance Parameters

This section describes the interference models used in the simulations and performance parameters calculated in the simulations.

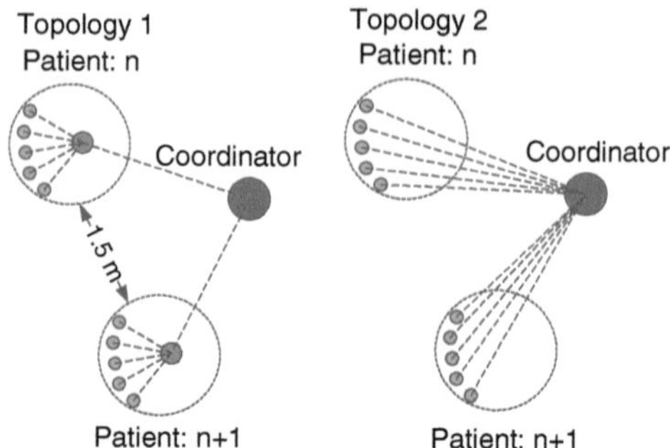

Fig. 3.12 Different network topologies used in the simulations

3.4.1 Network Topologies and Interference Model

Two different network topologies are simulated in order to investigate the effect of using intermediate router nodes on the network performance (Fig. 3.12). Topology 1 uses a router as an intermediate node between sensor nodes and coordinator node. The router node gathers data sent by the sensor nodes using a UWB receiver and transmits them to the coordinator node using a UWB transmitter. The router node uses a 433 MHz ISM band receiver to receive control messages related to router-coordinator interface from the coordinator node and transmits control messages related to router-sensor node interface using a narrowband transmitter operating in the same frequency band. Router nodes have the ability to store and forward data. Router nodes use the MAC protocol and super frame structure for its data communication with both sensor node side and the coordinator node side of the network. Data communication between router nodes and sensor nodes uses both CAP and CFP while data communication between router nodes and coordinator node uses only CFP with several GTS allocated per a router node depending on the data transmission requirement. Cluster tree routing [23], which is used for Zigbee is adapted for the use of UWB based data transmission and is implemented as the routing protocol in Topology 1. The motivation behind using a router as an intermediate node is to decentralize the coordination within the network by dividing it into sub networks. It also helps to optimize the power consumption in the sensor nodes. In Topology 2, sensor nodes directly communicate with the coordinator.

All the nodes are contained in a 10 m × 10 m Opnet simulation environment. The router nodes are kept at a distance of 0.5 m in Topology 1. An average separation of 1.5 m is assumed between the subnets in this topology. The router nodes are kept at an average distance of 1.5 m from the coordinator node. In Topology 2, each sensor node is placed at an average distance of 2 m from the coordinator node.

The interference between the subnets is minimized using two methods. As the first method, the pulse transmit power of the sensor nodes are set at a lower value, such that the power leakage between subnets is minimized. The power levels are further discussed under a following section. Secondly, each node is assigned with a unique address (see Sect. 3.3.5). In Topology 1, router nodes gather data from sensor nodes using the super frame structure described in Sect. 3.3.4. Due to the smaller number of sensor nodes that communicate with each router node, a larger inactive period is present in the super frame. This inactive period is utilized by the router nodes to map the data received from the sensor nodes into the super frame slots of the communication link between router nodes and coordinator node. The packet acknowledgement delay can be significantly reduced in this manner.

During data reception, the attenuated signal power from other simultaneous transmissions and simultaneous multipath receptions are added to the noise floor of the receiver (detected by the BER calculation at the parent node). It was observed from the simulations that the interference between narrowband signals and UWB signals are negligible. This is due to the large separation between the operational frequencies of those two types of signals.

During the simulation, sensor nodes are initiated in a random manner. Data rates used for sensor nodes are taken from Table 3.2. The data packets for continuous sensor nodes consist of nine bytes of physical overhead and 617 bytes of fragmented data payload, which is sent within one transmission slot of the super frame. Periodic sensors generate data packets with 6 bytes of overhead and 52 bits of data payload. For a fair assessment of both topologies, same number of sensor nodes is simulated in each case. Considering a realistic hospital scenario, five sensor nodes are attached to each patient out of which, one is a continuous implantable sensor node, one is a periodic implantable sensor node and others are periodic wearable sensor nodes. A maximum of seven patients are assumed to enter the room during the simulation time.[3] This number is decided based on the limitation of the GTS in Topology 2. More sensor nodes can be assigned in Topology 1, since the data can be buffered at the router before sending to the coordinator node.

For demonstrating the advantage of using a narrow band receiver in place of a UWB receiver in a sensor node, packet delay and energy consumption are analyzed for both cases. When a UWB receiver is used, the beacons are sent within the 35 µs guard period of the super frame structure. A 200 µs transmitter inactive period is added at the end of the super frame to allow for turnaround time and reception time. The parent nodes send feedback messages during this period. A 100 MHz PRF and 20 PPB is used for the receiver. It should be noted that the effective data rate is reduce due to the addition of the transmitter inactive time slot in this case. In the case of the sensor node with the narrow band receiver, the receiver is kept on during the whole sensor active period (throughout the period where the sensor is attempting to complete a transmission) in order to receive simultaneous downlink messages.

---

[3] This assumes that a hospital room accommodates up to seven patients for monitoring.

3.4.2 Transmit Power Allocation

Transmit power is a crucial factor in determining the pulse signal to noise ratio at the receiver. The maximum allowable indoor transmit power depends on duty cycle and PRF according the analysis in Sect. 3.3.1.The power limits for the implantable sensor nodes used in the simulations are set at a higher value than this limit, such that the indoor power limit just after the in-body propagation falls within the maximum allowable FBW transmit power limit. For example consider a continuous WCE sensor node in Topology 2. This is considered to be an implantable sensor node with an average implant depth of 80 mm. When transmitting at 2 PPB, this sensor node represents the maximum number of pulse transmissions within a duty cycled transmission slot in the network (10,000 pulses are sent within a 100 μs). Hence, the WCE sensor node transmitting at 2 PPB and a maximum allowable indoor FBW transmit power of 0.01 mW is used to calculate the maximum allowable indoor FBW transmit power for all the sensor nodes in the network. In this manner, all the sensor nodes transmit at an indoor FBW transmit power of 0.01 mW or less depending on their duty cycle.

In the case of the WCE sensor node, a maximum in-body path loss of 67.5 dB can be calculated using (3.1). Hence, the transmit power for this type of sensors are set to be 67.5 dB higher than the 0.01 mW value in order to obtain an indoor transmit power of 0.01 mW. For Topology 1, the transmit power for sensor nodes are reduced by 12 dB [calculated using (3.3)], in order to receive the same power at an average distance of 0.5 m in Topology 1 as the receive power at an average distance of 2 m for Topology 2. This minimizes the power leakage among subnets.

3.4.3 Performance Parameters

The following performance related metrics are calculated in the simulation:

$$PL = \frac{L}{S} \tag{3.14}$$

$$D = T1 - T2 \tag{3.15}$$

$$Normalised\ Throughput(\%) = \frac{R(\text{bps})}{C(\text{bps})} \times 100\ \% \tag{3.16}$$

$$E\left(\frac{\text{J}}{\text{bit}}\right) = \left(\frac{\sum_{i=0}^{K} \left(I(\text{A}) \times V(\text{V}) \times T_{tx-rx}(\text{s})\right)}{\sum_{i=0}^{K} B}\right) \tag{3.17}$$

where R (bps) is total data bit rate offered to the network by sensor nodes, C (bps) is the total network capacity that can be utilized by each sensor node type, PL is the

Table 3.3 Important simulation parameters

Parameter	Value
Total number of patients	7
Number of continuous implantable sensor nodes per patient	1
Number of periodic implantable sensor nodes per patient	1
Number of periodic wearable sensor nodes per patient	3
UWB frequency	3.5–4.5 GHz
Narrow band frequency	433.05–434.79 MHz

Table 3.4 Current/Power consumptions used for simulations

Parameter	Current/power consumption
UWB transmit	2 mW [2]
UWB receive	16 mA [2]
Narrowband receive	3.1 mA [6]
Sleep mode	0.2 mW

packet loss ratio, L is the total number of lost packets, S is the total number of sent packets, E is the consumed energy at a sensor node per useful data bit sent, I is the consumed current (A) of the sensor node, V (V) is the battery voltage, $T_{tx\text{-}rx}(\text{sec})$ is the sum of transmission time per data packet and reception time for acknowledgments /control packets at the sensor nodes, B is the total number of useful bits contained in above mentioned packets, K is the total number of packets sent, D is the packet acknowledgement delay for periodic traffic, $T1$ is the actual time at which the packet is acknowledged and $T2$ is the time at which a packet enters the transmission queue. The total network capacity (C) in throughput calculation is chosen such that it will represent the theoretical maximum throughput for each sensor type transmitting at a given moment. For example, if four continuous sensor nodes are transmitting simultaneously at a given instance, the total network capacity (C) for the continuous sensor nodes is chosen as 20 Mbps (5 Mbps × 4) considering their effective data rates. Important simulation parameters are listed in Table 3.3. The 433 MHz ISM band with Amplitude Shift Keying (ASK) is used for the narrow band feedback link. Narrow band specifications are chosen according to a commercial narrowband receiver [6] datasheet. Average current and power consumptions for electronics in transmitter and receiver models used in the simulations are shown in Table 3.4. The battery voltage is assumed to be 3 V.

3.5 Simulation Results

Simulation results for the analysis of various network parameters are obtained by running five simulations for each scenario and taking the average of each result. From the collected statistics, it was shown that the results might vary with ±4 % accuracy from the average value.

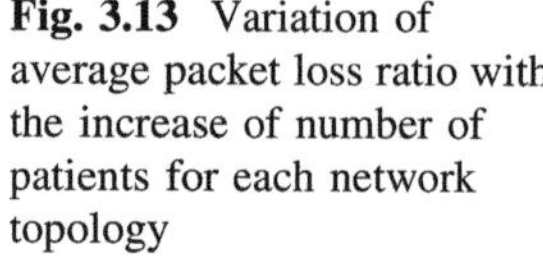

Fig. 3.13 Variation of average packet loss ratio with the increase of number of patients for each network topology

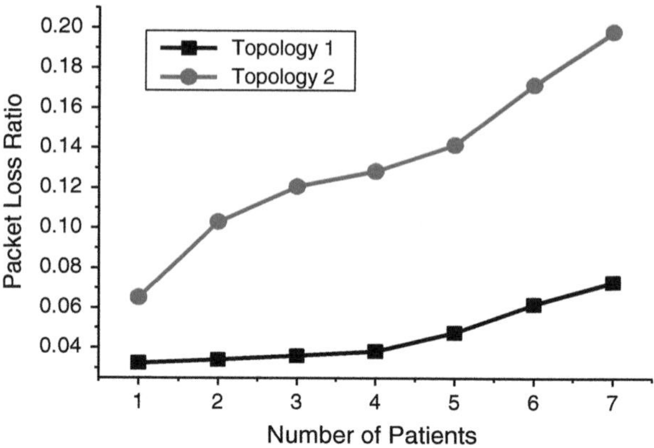

3.5.1 Packet Loss Ratio

Data transmitted over a WBAN is of utmost importance for a patient's health. Hence keeping the data loss at a minimum level is an important characteristic of a reliable WBAN. Packet loss ratio, which is determined by (3.14), is a good indicator of WBAN's susceptibility to data loss. Packet losses in a network occur due to various reasons, such as bad channel conditions and collisions. When the network is divided into sub networks, comparatively small number of sensor nodes contends for data transmission in a shared medium. Hence the number of collisions is reduced. In Fig. 3.13, it can be seen that the packet loss ratio for the network topology that uses a router as the intermediate node is lesser than that of Topology 2 where the sensor nodes directly coordinate with the coordinator without an intermediate node. In Topology 1, router nodes create a sub network with their child sensor nodes; hence, control of the system is more distributed than in Topology 2.

3.5.2 Average Packet Acknowledgement Delay

In a real life hospital scenario, it is expected that patient information be delivered as fast as possible to his life support systems. Hence packet delay of a WBAN should be kept in the minimum value possible. Average packet acknowledgement delay determined by (3.15) is an indicator of the time taken for a packet to be successfully transmitted and acknowledged. In the system described in this chapter, only periodic packets are acknowledged. Continuously transmitting sensor nodes are provided with guaranteed time slots; hence offering reliable transmission of packets. Data packets of continuously transmitting sensor nodes are not acknowledged. Instead, BER of continuous data is monitored in real time by the coordinator and a feedback is sent to sensor nodes only under degraded BER conditions. This technique helps to keep the packet delay at a minimum level for continuous sensor nodes.

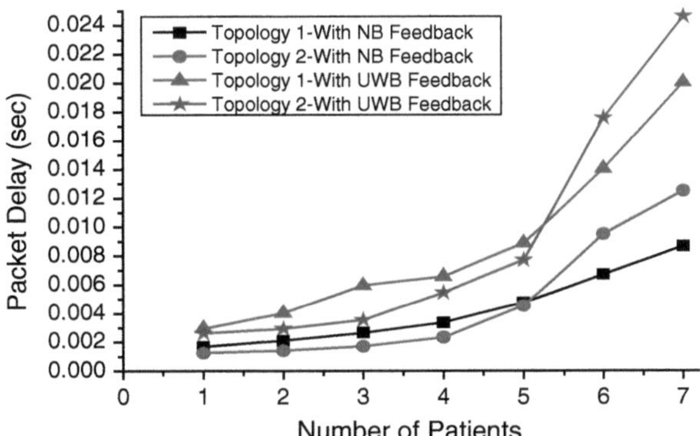

Fig. 3.14 Variation of the average packet acknowledgement delay (seconds) for periodic traffic with increasing number of patients for two topologies with and without narrow band feed back

Figure 3.14 shows that the packet acknowledgement delay of periodic sensor nodes in Topology 1 is lower than that of Topology 2 after the total number of active periodic sensor nodes increases more than 20 (five patients). Packet acknowledgment delay consists of the total time taken for queuing, medium access, inter frame space, packet transmission and acknowledgment reception. Medium access delay consists of time taken for allocating a time slot in the next frame during random access of periodic sensor nodes and back-off time taken in case of an unsuccessful time slot allocation. In Topology 1, only four periodic sensor nodes per router have to contend for sending data, while in Topology 2, all the periodic sensor nodes contend for a single shared medium. As the number of sensor nodes increases above a certain limit, the time delay that a sensor node is required to wait in order to send data through the shared medium will increase. It is observed from the simulations that both the allocation time and the back-off delay increase considerably in Topology 2 after total periodic sensor nodes increase above 20. It is also observed that contention in the links between the routers and the coordinator in Topology 1 is much lower than the contention level in the links between sensor nodes and coordinator in Topology 2. From the results it can be concluded that Topology 1 is more scalable than Topology 2.

With the introduction of narrow band feedback receiver, it is possible to do simultaneous transmission and reception at sensor nodes. Hence the time taken to switch from transmit state to a receive state when using a UWB transmitter and a UWB receiver in the sensor node can be eradicated by using a narrowband receiver. This is shown in the simulation results since the packet acknowledgement delay for the system with a narrow band feedback is lower than that of the system using UWB for both the transmitter and receiver.

3.5.3 Percentage Throughput

A WBAN should be capable of adjusting according to the varying load conditions in a hospital environment. Although most of the physiological signals are of

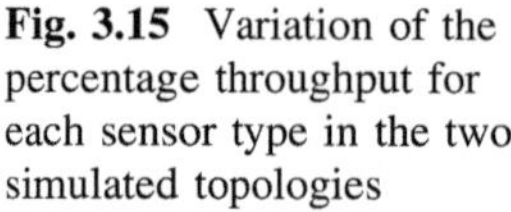

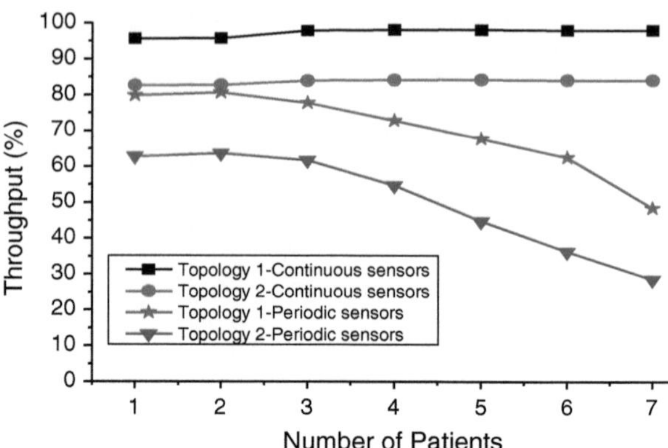

Fig. 3.15 Variation of the percentage throughput for each sensor type in the two simulated topologies

periodic nature, there is a possibility of sudden network load increase when a set of sensor nodes from a patient is turned on at the same time. This should not hinder the capability of the network to deliver the offered traffic from the sensor nodes. Since priority is given for critical physiological data, throughput of continuous data should be kept at a high value throughout the period of data transmission. Periodic signals like body temperature and heart rate are comparatively less time critical. Hence it is reasonable to allocate higher percentage of network capacity for continuous sensor nodes while dynamically varying the network capacity allocated for periodic sensors.

From Fig. 3.15 it can be seen that throughput percentage that can be achieved for both continuous and periodic traffic in Topology 1 is higher than that of Topology 2. Router nodes in Topology 1 offer channel resources only to their child nodes while in Topology 2, channel resources from coordinator node are shared between all the sensor nodes.

The throughput percentage for periodic data decreases with increasing sensor nodes in all two topologies. This is due to the fact that as the contention free traffic increases, timeslots available in the super frame for a contention based traffic decrease. The priority is given to continuous sensor nodes that transmit data in the contention free period.

3.5.4 Energy Consumption

A system with low power consumption will allow the battery powered sensor nodes in a WBAN to operate in an autonomous manner with less human intervention. From Fig. 3.16 it can be observed that the consumed energy at sensor nodes per useful bit is comparatively higher in Topology 2, which does not use an intermediate router. This power consumption value contains the power consumed for retransmissions as well. From the simulations it is observed that the number of retransmissions in Topology 1 is less than that of Topology 2 due to the distributed

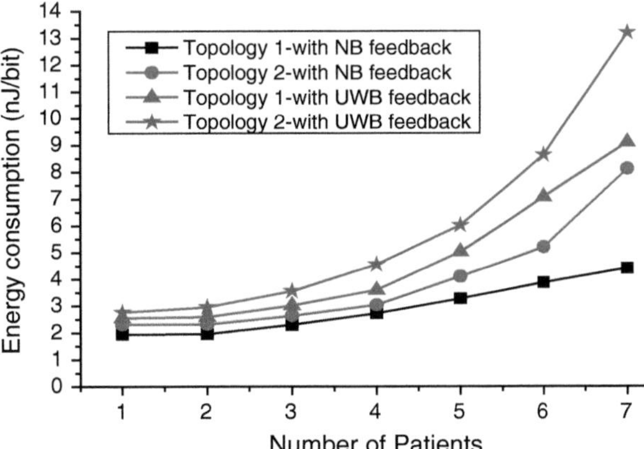

Fig. 3.16 Variation of consumed energy by a sensor node per useful data bit (in nJ) with increasing number of patients for two topologies and for sensor nodes with narrowband receivers and sensor nodes with UWB receivers

nature of the network. It should be noted that the router node is not required to be implantable or wearable; it can be kept at close proximity to its child sensor nodes. Both wearable and implantable sensor nodes should be designed to maximize the power savings, especially in health monitoring. For example, it is not practical to recharge a wearable ECG data transmitter frequently. It should be designed to operate without any intervention as long as possible. In the Topology 1, which uses a router, the transmit power of the sensor node can be kept at a minimum in order to achieve a given bit error rate (10^{-4} in this simulation). Hence the number of pulses that needs to be transmitted is comparatively lower than a sensor node in Topology 2. Since the channel characteristics at the receiver are fairly constant over short distance, the need of dynamically changing the number of pulses is lessen. Because of all these factors the sensor nodes in Topology 1 consume less power than sensor nodes of Topology 2. Energy consumption is also compared between sensor nodes with a narrow band receiver and a UWB receiver. From the obtained results it is obvious that the use of narrow band receiver reduces the power consumption significantly in the sensor node compared to the use of an UWB receiver. It should be noted that only transmitter and receiver power consumption figures are considered in these simulations and the power consumption of peripheral electronics are not considered since they affect all communication scenarios in a similar manner.

3.5.5 Comparison of Some Existing MAC Protocols

A comparison of the MAC protocol presented in this chapter with some of the existing MAC designs in the literature is shown in Table 3.5. The UWB MAC protocol discussed in this chapter demonstrates the ability to change the number of pulses per data bit in real-time. Thus, it is possible to cater variable data rate requirements while keeping the network utilization at a maximum level for high priority sensor nodes. The MAC protocol example presented in this chapter also

Table 3.5 Comparison of MAC protocols

Reference	Physical/ MAC layer	Presence of adaptive data rate	Priority driven traffic	Maximum reported per sensor node data throughput	Maximum reported air interface raw data rate	Maximum reported packet delay	Minimum energy consumption
[24]	UWB/IEEE 802.15.4a	–	–	3.35 Mbps (in the presence of 32 simultaneous transmissions)	8 Mbps	–	–
[25]	4 GHz IR-UWB/ PSMA, Slotted Aloha	–	Yes	3 kbps [ECG sensor with Slotted Aloha (in the presence of 50 simultaneous transmission)]	850 kbps	–	0.07 µJ/bit (for 5 simultaneous ECG sensors, Tx. Power = 20 mW, Rx. Power = 116 mW, including interface electronics)
[26]	ISM /IEEE 802.15.6	–	–	700 kbps (2.4 GHz band for a payload size of 250 bytes with no simultaneous transmissions)	–	30.78 ms in 420-450 MHz band for a payload size of 250 bytes with no simultaneous transmissions.	–
[27]	ISM/ Raccoon	–	Yes	4 kbps (ECG ch1 when 10 WBAN s with 6 sensors in each WBAN transmitting simultaneously)	48 kbps	1.5 s when 10 WBAN s with 6 sensors in each WBAN transmitting simultaneously	2.5 mW/bit (for 1 WBAN with 6 sensors, Tx power = 31.2 mW and Rx. Power = 27.3 mW, including interface electronics)

(continued)

Table 3.5 (continued)

Reference	Physical/ MAC layer	Presence of adaptive data rate	Priority driven traffic	Maximum reported per sensor node data throughput	Maximum reported air interface raw data rate	Maximum reported packet delay	Minimum energy consumption
[28]	IR-UWB/ IEEE 802.15.4a	–	–	~10 kbps (in the presence of 5 simultaneous transmissions)	1 Mbps	3.1 ms (25 simultaneous sensors)	–
Dual-band WBAN (This design)	4 GHz IR-UWB/ Random access	Yes	Yes	5 Mbps (WCE sensors,in the presence of 35 simultaneous transmissions)	5 Mbps	8 ms (35 simultaneous sensors-Topology 1), 12 ms (35 simultaneous sensors-Topology 2)	2 nJ/bit (for 5 sensors, Tx power = 2 mW, Rx power = 3 V@3.1 mA, without considering interface electronics)

provides guaranteed delivery mechanism for high priority traffic. This MAC algorithm is a good MAC design example that has incorporated the physical layer properties of IR-UWB, such as number of pulses per data bit, and burst transmission period, which can be considered as a unique feature of this design. A scalable data rate of up to 5 Mbps can be achieved using this MAC protocol depending on the number of pulses per bit and pulse transmission interval. Also it is possible to operate the sensor nodes at the maximum allowable transmit power by selecting the burst transmission slot as mentioned in Sect. 3.3. The maximum total delay demonstrated in the simulations is in the range of 8–12 ms for this design. The power consumption for a sensor node employing a UWB transmitter and a narrow band receiver ranges from 2 to 4 nJ/bit. This value is obtained by considering the power consumption of transmitter and receiver without any additional interface electronics required for the operation of the sensor node (e.g. micro-controllers, ADC and front-end amplifiers.

3.6 Conclusion

In this chapter a number of unique techniques have been presented for UWB based WBAN systems. First of all, a dual band (UWB transmit and narrow band receive) physical layer is discussed for WBAN sensor nodes to achieve a power consumption lower than the current state of art technologies while maintaining a good QoS. The technique has been evaluated for a WBAN scheme that is formed by two networks to enable remote monitoring of a multi-human body environment. Details of a MAC protocol is discussed and studied for real-time implementation of WBAN systems. Furthermore, the MAC protocol is designed to dynamically vary the number of pulses per bit in the UWB transmission according to the received signal condition. Performance is analyzed by comparing network metrics presented in the results. From the results it can be observed that using a router as an intermediate node improves the data transmission within a WBAN. It is also shown that we can minimize the power consumption and packet delays for a UWB-based WBAN sensor node using a narrow band receiver. Hardware implementation of sensor nodes considering the MAC protocol given in this chapter and real-time measurement results are presented in Chap. 6.

References

1. K.M. Thotahewa, J.Y. Khan, M.R. Yuce, Power efficient ultra wide band based wireless body area networks with narrowband feedback path. IEEE Trans. Mobile Commun. (to appear)
2. M.R. Yuce, T.N. Dissanayake, H.C. Keong, in *Wideband Technology for Medical Detection and Monitoring, Recent Advances in Biomedical Engineering*, ed. by G.R Naik (InTech, Florida, 2009). ISBN: 978-953-307-004-9

3. H.C. Keong, M.R. Yuce, Analysis of a multi-access scheme and asynchronous transmit-only UWB for Wireless Body Area Networks. The 31st annual international conference of the IEEE engineering in medicine and biology society (EMBC'09), pp. 6906–6909, 2009

4. H.C. Keong, K.M. Thotahewa, M.R. Yuce, Transmit-only ultra wide band (UWB) body sensors and collision analysis. IEEE Sens. J. **13**, 1949–1958 (2013)

5. K.M. Silva, M.R Yuce, J.Y. Khan, Network topologies for dual band (UWB—transmit and Narrow Band- receive) Wireless Body Area Network, in *Proceedings of the ACM/IEEE Body Area Networks (BodyNets)*, 7–8 Nov 2011

6. http://www.rfm.com/products/data/rx5500.pdf, 2013

7. http://www.mathworks.com, 2013

8. http://www.opnet.com, 2013

9. M.R. Yuce, Ho Chee Keong, M. Chae, Wideband communication for implantable and wearable systems. IEEE Trans. Microw. Theory Tech. **57**(2), 2597–2604 (2009)

10. A. Ridolfi, M.Z. Win, Ultrawide bandwidth signals as shot noise: a unifying approach. IEEE J. Sel. Areas Commun. **24**(4), 899–905 (2006)

11. A. Khaleghi, R. Chavez-Santiago, X. Liang, I. Balasingham, V.C.M. Leung, T.A. Ramstad, On ultra wideband channel modeling for in-body communications, in *5th IEEE International Symposium on Wireless Pervasive Computing*, pp. 140–145, 2010

12. IEEE P802.15-02/240-SG3a, Empirically Based Statistical Ultra-Wideband Channel Model

13. IEEE P802.15-02/490r1-SG3a, Channel Modeling Sub-committee Report Final, February 2003

14. R.J. Punnoose, P.V. Nikitin, D.D. Stancil, Efficient simulation of ricean fading within a packet simulator. IEEE Veh. Technol. Conf. **2**, 764–767 (2000)

15. FCC 02-48 (First Report and Order), 2002

16. R.J. Fontana, E.A. Richley, Observations on low data rate, short pulse UWB systems. IEEE international conference on ultra-wideband, pp. 334–338, 2007

17. FCC 05-58: Petition for waiver of the part 15 UWB regulations. Filed by the multi-band OFDM Alliance Special Interest Group, ET Docket 04-352, March 11, 2005

18. H. Chee Keong, M.R. Yuce, Transmit only UWB body area network for medical applications. Asia Pacific microwave conference, pp. 2200–2203, 2009

19. K. Witrisal, G. Leus, G.J.M. Janssen, M. Pausini, F. Troesch, T. Zasowski, J. Romme, Noncoherent ultra-wideband systems. IEEE Signal Process. Mag. **26**(4), 48, 66 (2009)

20. I. Guvenc, H. Arslan, S. Gezici, H. Kobayashi, Adaptation of two types of processing gains for UWB impulse radio wireless sensor networks. IET Commun. **1**(6), 1280, 1288 (2007)

21. IEEE-802.15.4-2006, Part 15.4: wireless medium access control (MAC) and physical layer (PHY) specifications for low-rate wireless personal area networks (LR-WPANs). Standard, IEEE

22. IEEE-802.15.4a-2007, Part 15.4: Wireless medium access control (MAC) and physical layer (PHY) specifications for low-rate wireless personal area networks (LR-WPANs): amendment to add alternate PHY. Standard, IEEE

23. J. Sun, Z. Wang, H. Wang, X. Zhang, Research on routing protocols based on ZigBee network. Third international conference on intelligent information hiding and multimedia signal processing, vol. 1, pp. 639–642, 2007

24. J.Y. Le Boudec, R. Merz, B. Radunovic, J. Widmer, DCCMAC: A decentralized MAC protocol for 802.15.4a-Like UWB mobile Ad-Hoc networks based on dynamic channel coding. Broadnets, 2004

25. L. Kynsijarvi, L. Goratti, R. Tesi, J. Iinatti, M. Hamalainen, Design and performance of contention based MAC protocols in WBAN for medical ICT using IR-UWB, in *IEEE 21st International Symposium on Personal, Indoor and Mobile Radio Communications Workshops*, pp. 107–111, 26–30 Sept 2010

26. S. Ullah, M. Chen, K. Kwak, Throughput and delay analysis of IEEE 802.15.6-based CSMA/CA protocol. J. Med. Syst. **36**(6), 3875–3891 (2012)

27. S. Cheng, C. Huang, C. Tu, RACOON: a multiuser QoS design for mobile wireless body area networks. J. Med. Syst. **35**(5), 1277–1287 (2011)
28. L. De Nardis, G. Giancola, M.-G.Di Benedetto, Performance analysis of uncoordinated medium access control in low data rate UWB networks. 2nd International Conference on Broadband Networks, vol. 2, pp. 1129–1135, 7-7 Oct 2005

Chapter 4
Hardware Architectures
for IR-UWB-Based Transceivers

Abstract Impulse Radio-Ultra-wideband (IR-UWB) is an attractive wireless technology for Wireless Body Area Network (WBAN) applications. Low power transmitter design and low complexity hardware implementation present the possibility of developing sensor nodes with small form factors with high data rate capability. A UWB transceiver is the core unit required in a UWB based WBAN system that provide wireless communications. It determines critical properties of the WBAN, such as data rate and power consumption. This chapter focuses on the hardware implementation of UWB based sensor nodes for WBAN applications. Different realizations of UWB transceiver architectures are described and a critical analysis of their suitability for WBAN applications is presented. In addition, different UWB pulse generation techniques are discussed.

Keywords UWB transmitters · UWB receivers · UWB pulse generation · Hardware implementation · Base band pulse generators · Up-conversion pulse generators · Coherent UWB receivers · Non-coherent UWB receivers · AcR receivers · Transmit-only hardware

4.1 Introduction

UWB transceivers are the main building blocks of any UWB sensor node. UWB transmitters are simple in design and consume a smaller amount of power compared to their narrow band counterparts. An IR-UWB transmitter design consists of an UWB pulse generator. IR-UWB pulse generators can be divided into subcategories, such as base band pulse generators and up-conversion pulse generators.

IR-UWB receivers are more complex in design and consume larger amount of power than IR-UWB transmitters. This poses a challenge to use IR-UWB technology in low-power WBAN devices. It is possible to investigate alternative approaches that lead to incorporating advantages provided by IR-UWB transmitters, while avoiding the disadvantages of using IR-UWB receivers in wearable and

K. M. S. Thotahewa et al., *Ultra Wideband Wireless Body Area Networks*, 67
DOI: 10.1007/978-3-319-05287-8_4,
© Springer International Publishing Switzerland 2014

implantable hardware platforms. IR-UWB receivers can be divided into two major categories: non-coherent receivers and coherent receivers. Suitability of these two types of UWB receivers largely depends on the nature of the application.

This chapter investigates the implementation of UWB based transceivers for WBAN applications. Different design methodologies reported in the literature for the implementation of UWB transmitters and receivers are discussed in this chapter highlighting their advantages and disadvantages.

4.2 UWB Transmitter Design Techniques

The UWB transmitter lies at the core of a UWB based sensor node. Unlike in the case of the narrow band transmitters, the Radio Frequency (RF) portion of the UWB transmitters does not dictate the overall power consumption. Hence, care has to be taken in order to minimize the power consumption of the rest of the transmitter circuitry. This section will analyze some common transmitter design techniques that are available in the literature.

A UWB transmitter design starts with a narrow UWB pulse generator. The earlier versions of the UWB pulse generators used Step Recovery Diodes (SRD) in order to generate the pulses and Schottky diodes for pulse shaping. In this technique, the SRD creates a voltage step function with a very short rise time [1, 2]. A delayed version of this step function is also created by making the step function to propagate through a transmission line. The original step function is combined with the delayed version of itself in order to make a narrow UWB pulse. There are several drawbacks in this method of pulse generation that make this technique less attractive for WBAN applications. The length of the transmission line used in order to obtain the delayed version of the pulse is quite large; hence it results in a large form factor in the circuit design. The pulse generation method is very sensitive to the reflections that may occur in the wave propagation paths; hence the operation of the circuit can be largely affected even by a small fabrication fault. The amplitudes of the pulses that can be generated by this method are limited to few hundreds of millivolts (mV) [1]. Hence it requires extensive amplification before transmitting through a wireless link. However, this method provides the basis for most of the modern UWB pulse generation techniques; that is the combining of a waveform and its delayed version in order to generate narrow pulses.

UWB pulse generators can be categorized into three major categories; namely (1) base band pulse generators, (2) up-conversion pulse generators and (3) waveform synthesis pulse generators. These three pulse generation techniques are further described in the following sections.

4.2.1 Base Band UWB Pulse Generators

In this approach, a base band pulse is generated initially in the form of a rectangular pulse [3–6]. The square base band pulse provides signal with a wide spectrum. However, initial base band pulse does not comply with the FCC spectrum requirements. Hence, a filtering stage is used in order to shape the pulse spectrum, such that it complies with the FCC spectral mask. This approach is shown in Fig. 4.1.

In base band pulse generators, the square pulse and its delayed version is passed through an XOR gate, forming an edge combining circuit. The narrow square pulses formed by the XOR output are then filtered using either a passive Band Pass Filter (BPF) [3, 5] or a Finite Impulse Response (FIR) based filter [7]. The square pulses that form the input to the XOR gate can be obtained either using the input data waveform itself [8, 9], through a flip-flop arrangement [5] or using a separate clock waveform [4].

An example pulse generator that uses a clock as the square wave signal source is depicted in Fig. 4.2 [10]. The use of an 'AND' gate after the 'XOR' gate creates IR-UWB pulses at every positive edge of the clock signal. The UWB pulses are then modulated with the data signal using another 'AND' gate.

The base band pulse generation method provides advantages in terms of simplicity in design. It avoids the complexities of directly generating the UWB pulses that comply with the FCC spectrum requirements. A significant portion of the power spectrum of the square wave has to be filtered in order to bring the UWB pulse spectrum into the target frequency range. This results in significant power loss. The amplitude of the UWB pulse spectrum after the BPF stage is often lower than the FCC spectral mask. Thus, a power amplification stage may be needed after the BPF in order to use the maximum allowable spectral amplitude. The use of a power amplifier further increases power consumption of the UWB transmitter.

4.2.2 Up-Conversion-Based UWB Pulse Generators

The up-conversion method uses a mixer to up convert the frequency of the base band pulses into the target frequency range. Both rectangular [11] and triangular [12] pulses can be used as the base band pulse stream. Up-conversion of the pulses eliminates the requirement of a base band pulse with a wide spectrum, such as a square pulse in order to generate the final UWB pulse stream. Hence a triangular pulse stream is more suitable as the basis of the pulse generation. The power spectrum of the triangular pulses has suppressed side lobes, compared to that of the rectangular pulses. Hence the power loss that might occur by using a square wave pulse as the base band pulse can be reduced. However, it should be noted that although the triangular pulse generation techniques are easily achievable in CMOS IC based designs, the rectangular pulse based approach is the most convenient

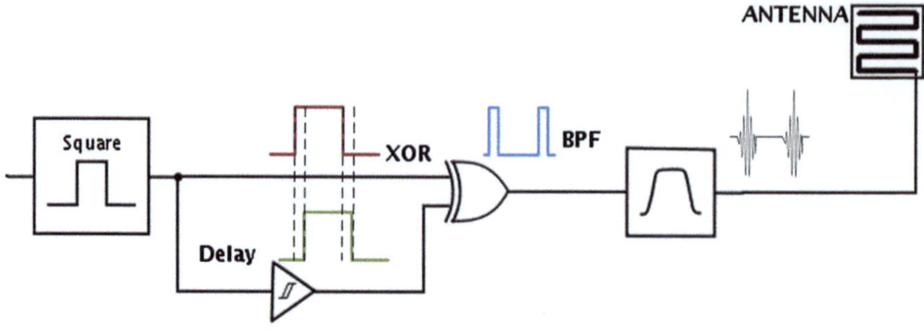

Fig. 4.1 Base band pulse generation approach

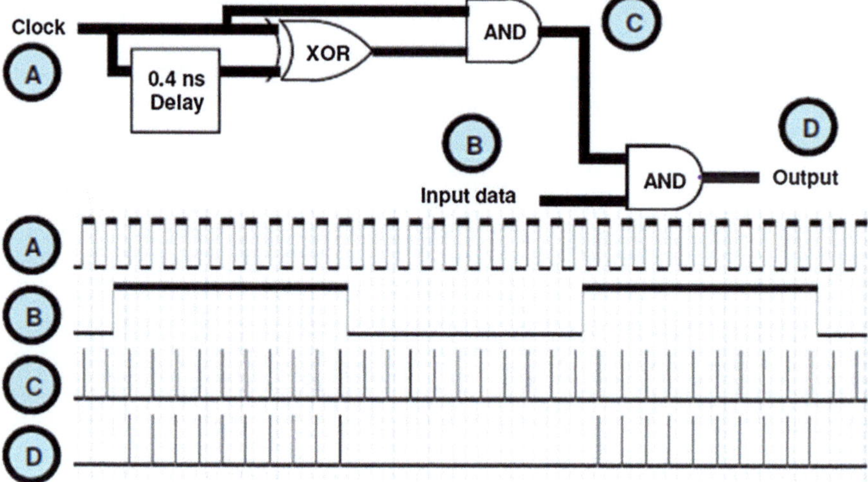

Fig. 4.2 An example pulse generation circuit [10], IEEE copyright

approach for the development of UWB pulse generators using off-the-shelf components. The up-conversion UWB pulse generation technique described in [12] is shown in Fig. 4.3.

In this method, the triangular pulse is generated using an integration circuit in combination with an inverter. The triangular pulse generator in fed with a Pulse Position Modulated (PPM) data waveform. The integration happens at the rising and falling edges of the data waveform. The amplitude of the baseband triangular pulse can be determined by the threshold of the integrator. The baseband triangular pulse is then up-converted into the higher frequencies using a mixer. The ring activation circuit activates the oscillator only when a pulse is present, hence it reduces the overall energy consumption of the circuit.

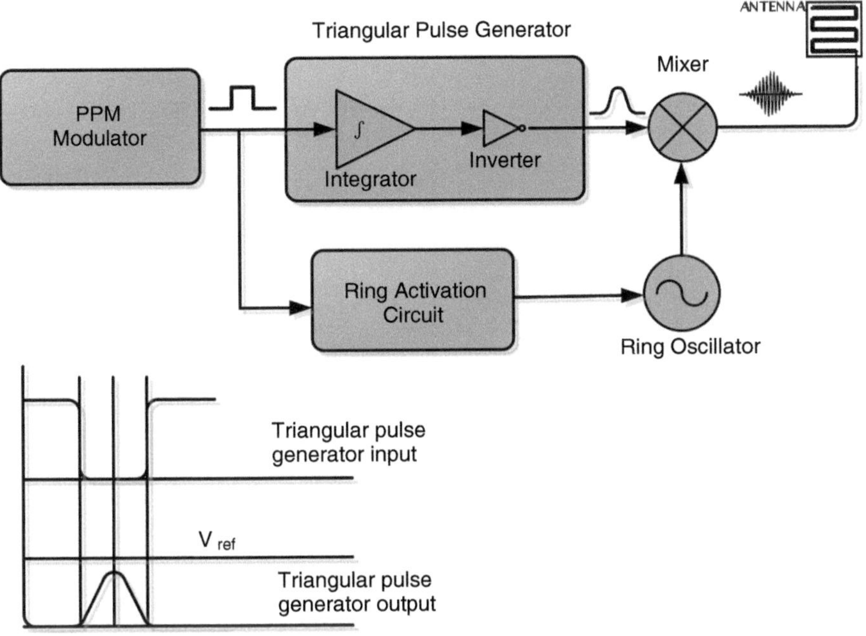

Fig. 4.3 Triangular pulse based up-conversion pulse generator

The use of an integrator for triangular pulse generation increases the power consumption of the circuit. A more efficient triangular pulse generation mechanism using logic gates is described in [13], where the triangular pulse is generated by edge combining the rising and falling edges of a square wave with an inverted version of itself.

The up-conversion pulse generation technique has the same advantages as the base band pulse generation technique. Additionally, the spectral shape of the final pulse can be determined in the base band domain in this method. Consequently, baseband pulse shaping techniques can be applied to this method rather than shaping the pulses at high frequencies. Hence, this approach minimizes the use of the power hungry RF components. However, this method also suffers from the relatively high power consumption in the mixer and the oscillator.

4.2.3 Waveform Synthesis (Pulse Shaping) Techniques for UWB Pulse Generators

In some UWB pulse generators, UWB pulses are directly synthesized in the targeted frequency range using pulse-shaping techniques. Unlike base band pulse generators, this type of UWB pulse generators do not use a base band pulse stream to filter out the signals with spectral portion at the target frequency range. It uses

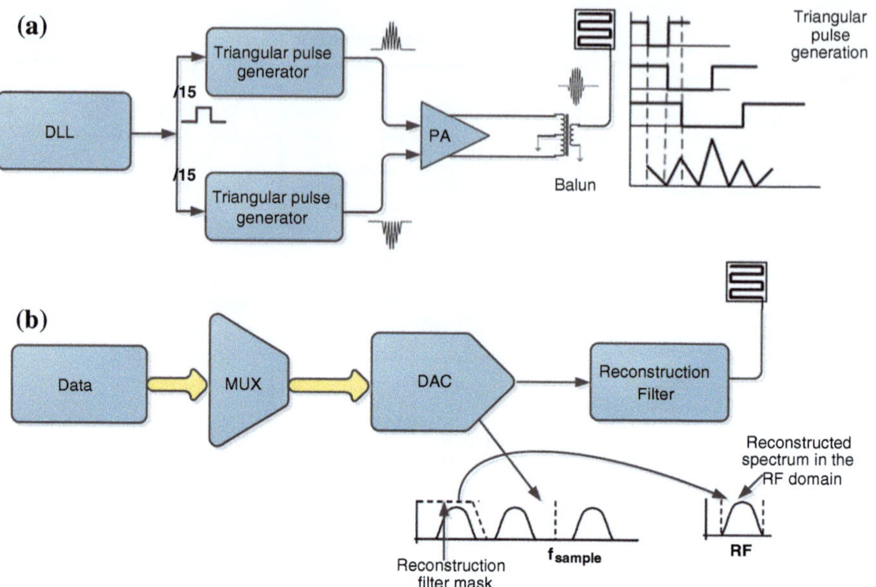

Fig. 4.4 Waveform synthesis UWB pulse generators **a** triangular pulse synthesis **b** DAC based pulse synthesis

waveform synthesis techniques to directly synthesize UWB pulses such that they directly fall within the target frequency range without using any filtering techniques. Direct synthesis of the UWB pulses can be realized using several methods. The methods shown in [14, 15] generate triangular pulses in the RF domain. A fully digital implementation of a triangular UWB pulse generator is described in [14]. In this method, the triangular pulses are generated by combining the edges of several square pulses created using a Delay Locked Loop (DLL) (Fig. 4.4a). The pulse shape can be digitally controlled by varying the delay of the original square pulses; hence, it is preferred over the analog pulse generation techniques for low power applications. Power amplification is applied for the negative and positive triangular pulses separately. Finally, the pulses are combined using a balun. This method provides more controllability over the pulse generation at the cost of increased hardware complexity.

A less complex, logic gate based triangular pulse generation technique is presented in [15]. In this method, the triangular pulses generated using a combination of XOR gates are used to periodically switch a voltage controlled ring oscillator. In this manner it is possible to generate the triangular UWB pulses in the RF domain. Since the oscillator operates only during the presence of a pulse, this method reduces the power wastage due to the continuous operation of local oscillators in the other methods.

A Digital to Analog Converter (DAC) based direct UWB pulse synthesis approach is demonstrated in [16] (Fig. 4.4b). This technique uses a high speed DAC in order to synthesize accurate UWB pulse in the RF domain. This method overlooks the precision in pulse generation, hence the achievable controllability in the pulse spectrum over the hardware complexity. The main drawback of this approach is that the DAC has to operate at very high sampling rates (in the order of 10 Gsps) in order to generate the UWB pulses. This is not only challenging for the implementation of the DAC, but also the input data stream has to operate at very high rates; hence it demands the use of high speed logic circuits. In general, the waveform synthesis UWB pulse generation method is suitable for on-chip implementations using advanced technologies such as CMOS due to the requirement of the high precision in circuit implementation.

4.3 UWB Receiver Design Techniques

Due to the short pulse width and low power of the signal, front-end circuitry for the UWB receiver is complex in design and has high power consumption. An Analog to Digital Converter (ADC) in a UWB receiver requires a large input bandwidth and a high sampling rate. For example ADC12D1800 [17] by National Semiconductors has 3.5 Giga samples per second sampling rate and an input bandwidth of 1.75 GHz, but it consumes 4.4 W of power which is not suitable for battery powered UWB sensor design. Although the ADC has been brought close to the antenna with the evolution of the front-end circuitry for narrow band systems, it is not considered as a suitable technique for UWB systems. The fully digital implementations of the UWB receivers require precise synchronization of nanosecond scale narrow UWB pulses and resolving numerous multipath components of the received UWB signals [18].

UWB receivers are of two types: non-coherent receivers and coherent receivers. These two receiver architectures are discussed in following sections.

4.3.1 Non-Coherent UWB Receivers

Non-coherent UWB receivers can be further sub-divided into two categories: Energy Detection (ED) receivers and Autocorrelation (AcR) receivers. ED UWB receiver architectures are discussed in [19, 20]. In this receiver type, a squaring device is used to correlate the received UWB signal with itself. This can be achieved by operating a MOSFET in the saturation region. Block diagram of the receiver described in [20] is shown in Fig. 4.5. The ED UWB receivers do not require channel estimation; hence hardware complexity is greatly reduced. This leads to superior performance in terms of power consumption. However the Signal-to-Noise Ratio (SNR) of this type of receivers is inferior to other types of UWB receivers mainly due to use of the noisy received signal as the template signal. Also, the receiver performance degrades rapidly in an environment with a large number of interferers.

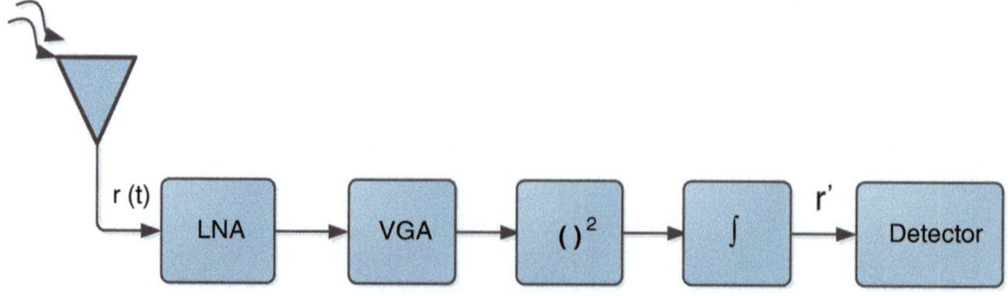

Fig. 4.5 An energy detection non-coherent UWB receiver

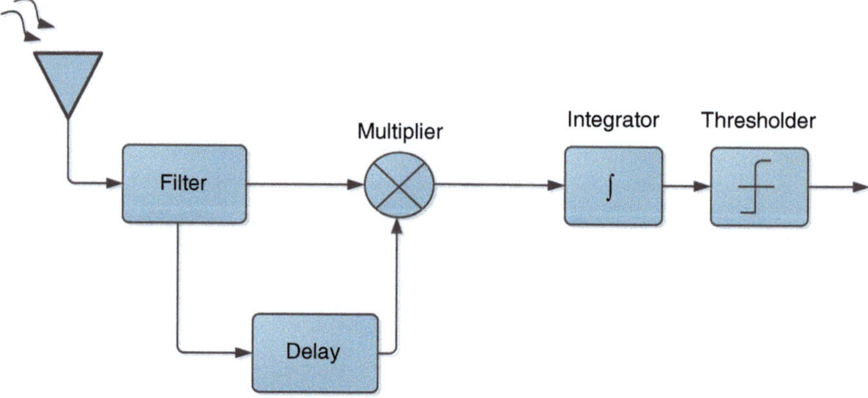

Fig. 4.6 An autocorrelation non-coherent UWB receiver

AcR receivers use a delay path and a multiplier circuit instead of the squarer circuit in the energy detection receiver. The operation of AcR receivers is based on the use of a reference pulse that is transmitted by the transmitter in order to correlate with the data modulated pulses that follow the reference pulse. The reference pulse that is transmitted prior to every data modulated pulse is delayed using a delay line, and is used as the signal template for the data reception that follows. The channel information embedded in the reference pulse improves the performance of the receiver by reducing the Inter Symbol Interference (ISI). Basic diagram of an AcR receiver is shown in Fig. 4.6. Performance of AcR receivers is discussed in [21, 22]. The main drawback of an AcR receiver is the requirement of a precise delay line. It also suffers from performance deterioration due to the use of a noisy template.

The BER performance of both the ED and the AcR receivers depend on the integration window time, which determines the amount of signal energy gathered during the integration period [18]. Further, it has shown in [18] that the ED receiver outperforms the AcR receiver in terms of BER for OOK and Binary Pulse Position Modulation (BPPM) schemes. Results in [23] demonstrates that the ED receiver is more power efficient than the AcR receiver.

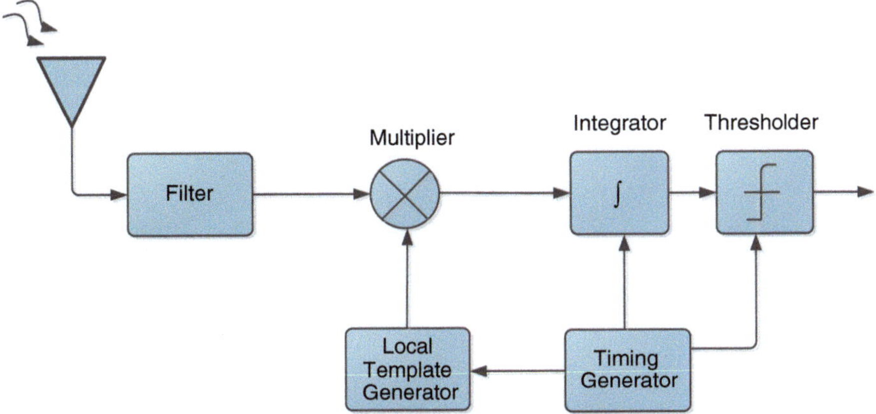

Fig. 4.7 A coherent UWB receiver

4.3.2 Coherent UWB Receivers

In a coherent receiver, correlation is performed between the received waveform
and a locally generated template of the waveform. It requires having a good
estimate of the channel, and a template generation mechanism, which makes it
complex in design and high power consuming. The development of an optimum
coherent receiver is demonstrated in [24]. Figure 4.7 depicts a basic block diagram
of the optimum coherent receiver architecture. The template generated at the local
template generator of the optimum coherent receiver is closely matched to the
transmitted signal. It also has to perform channel estimation in order to compensate for the presence of multipath components. This results in increased design
complexity and high power consumption.

Coherent rake receivers use energy of precise multipath components of the UWB
signal in order to reconstruct the original waveform [25]. This type of coherent
receivers requires large number of rake fingers due to the high temporal resolution of
the UWB signals. Performance of both types of coherent receivers deteriorates with
timing jitters and synchronization errors [26]. Performance of coherent receivers is
compared with that of a non-coherent receiver in [27, 28], which show that better
accuracy can be obtained in coherent receivers at the cost of high circuit complexity
and high power consumption. It has been shown in [28] that a non- coherent receiver
will perform better than a coherent receiver for timing jitter values above 18 ps.

4.4 UWB Sensor Node Designs

While many publications present the implementation of UWB transmitters in
Integrated Circuits (IC), only few publications present the full implementation of
UWB based sensor platforms that should other peripheral electronics, such as

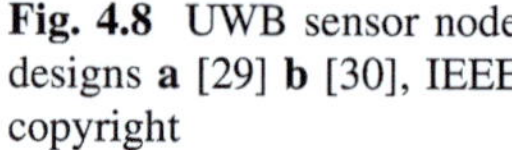

Fig. 4.8 UWB sensor node designs **a** [29] **b** [30], IEEE copyright

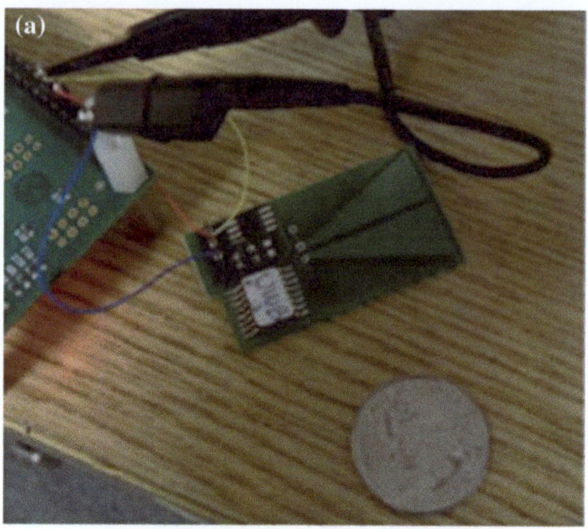

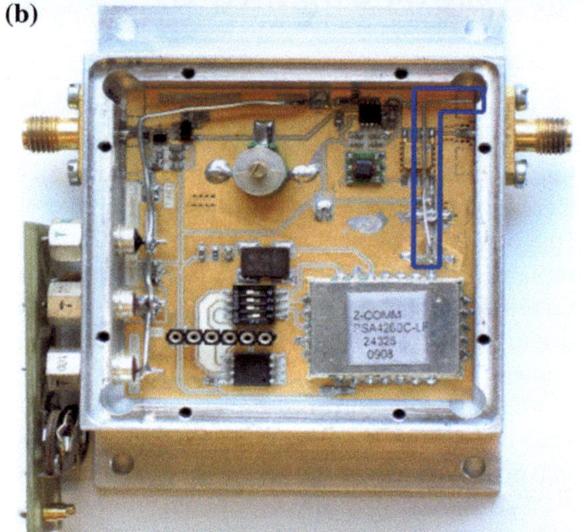

micro-controllers, sensor front-end circuits, receiver back-end processing units and matching circuits. This section presents some of the full implementations of UWB based sensor nodes that can be found in literature.

An UWB sensor node built based on a UWB pulse generator IC is presented in [29] (Fig. 4.8a). In this design, switched voltage control ring oscillator approach is used in order to generate the UWB pulses. The data is fed into the circuit using a Field Programmable Gate Array (FPGA) and is modulated using the pulse stream generated by the aforementioned pulse generation technique. This work also presents the implementation of a UWB antenna on the same Printed Circuit Board

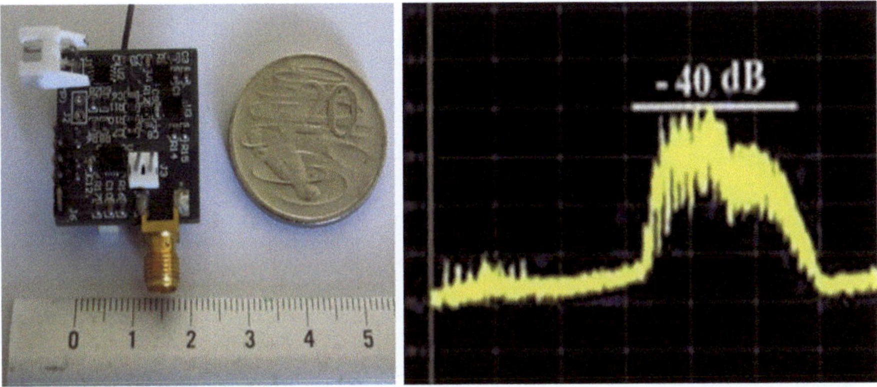

Fig. 4.9 Amplifier based UWB sensor node design and transmit spectrum

(PCB). This sensor node is not fully integrated for independent operation as the data and the control signals have to be generated using an external FPGA.

A UWB transmitter developed using off-the-shelf components is presented in [30]. In this method, narrow square pulses are generated in the base band domain using a series of comparators. The RF pulses are generated by mixing these narrow pulses with a high frequency signal generated using a phase locked loop. The power consumption of this circuit is 660 mW; hence it is not suitable for power stringent UWB applications.

A transmit-only UWB sensor node design is presented in [31, 32] (Fig. 4.9). Its main operational blocks are depicted in Fig. 4.10. The sensor nodes are assembled on a four layer PCB with dimensions of 27 mm (L) $\times$ 25 mm (W) $\times$ 1.5 mm (H), which is sufficiently compact for the use in a wearable WBAN node. This sensor node is designed using an amplifier based hardware architecture. In this design, the narrow base band pulses are filtered using a BPF with a pass-band of 3.5–4.5 GHz. The UWB pulses are then amplified using a wideband low noise amplifier (LNA) to meet the −41.3 dBm transmission power level. This amplifier has been included to guarantee that the amplitudes of the UWB pulses are sufficient to provide a targeted coverage by a WBAN application.

The power spectrum of the UWB pulses generated using this sensor node is shown in Fig. 4.11. This power spectrum consists of several frequency lobes spread throughout the UWB bandwidth. The amplitudes of these frequency lobes decrease towards the upper part of the UWB spectrum. The UWB sensor node is designed to transmit UWB signals in the band of 3.5–4.5 GHz. As shown in Fig. 4.11a, the amplitude of the frequency lobe within the 3.5–4.5 GHz band is well below the maximum allowable power level by the FCC (−41.3 dBm/MHz). This sensor node design employs two amplifier stages in order to boost the power level of the transmitted UWB signal within the band of 3.5–4.5 GHz (as marked in Fig. 4.11) while containing the power level within the FCC spectral mask.

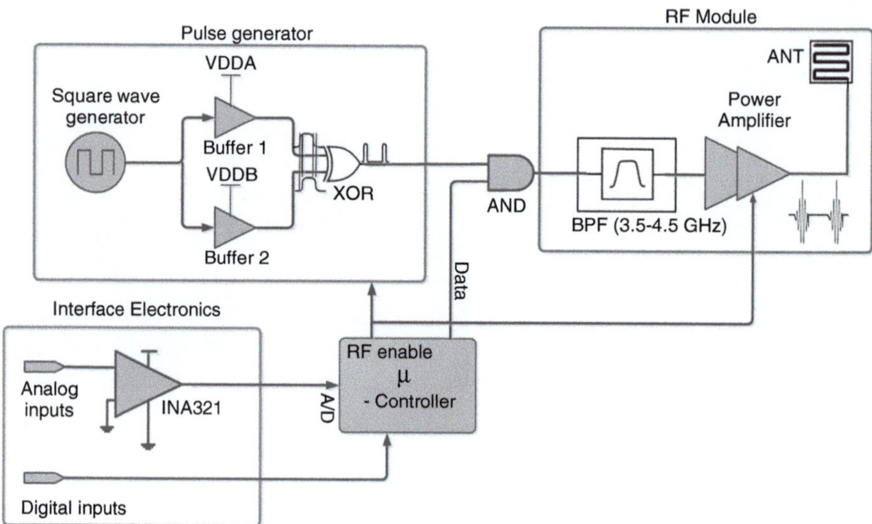

Fig. 4.10 Amplifier based UWB sensor node design

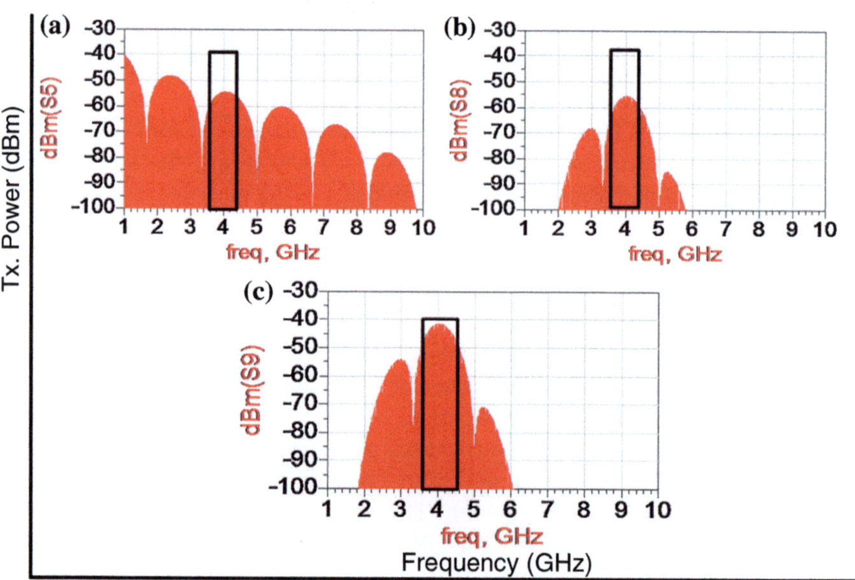

Fig. 4.11 Frequency spectrum of amplifier based sensor node at **a** pulse generator output **b** band pass filter (3.5–4.5 GHz) output, and **c** amplifier output

4.5 Conclusion

This chapter gives a brief introduction for some of the commonly used transceiver architectures used in UWB hardware implementations. Three types of pulse generators used in UWB transmitter developments are discussed, namely: base band pulse generators, up-conversion based pulse generators and waveform synthesis pulse generators. Among these three pulse generation methods, up-conversion based pulse generation method provides significant advantages in terms of low power consumption and simple design. This method can be considered as a suitable design technique for UWB transmitters. Waveform synthesis pulse generators generate pulses directly in the intended frequency range of an UWB application without using an intermediate base band stage. They are more complex in design compared to the up-conversion method. This type of pulse generators can be considered as a suitable design technique for IC based power efficient UWB hardware designs.

UWB receivers are inherently complex in design compared to UWB transmitters. This is mainly because of the fact that UWB receivers have to receive low power narrow UWB signals and have to perform functions, such as precise synchronization of narrow UWB pulses. There are two main realizations of UWB receivers: coherent receivers and non-coherent receivers. Non-coherent UWB receivers are better suited for WBAN applications mainly due to less complex hardware design and low power consumption. Out of the non-coherent UWB receivers, ED receivers are preferable over the AcR receivers, especially for short-range applications where a strong Line-Of-Sight (LOS) is present. This is mainly due to the fact that AcR receivers require the synthesis of precise delay lines, which leads way to complex hardware synthesis.

References

1. H. Jeongwoo, N. Cam, A new ultra-wideband, ultra-short monocycle pulse generator with reduced ringing. IEEE Microw. Wirel. Compon. Lett. **12**, 206–208 (2002)
2. L. Jeong-Soo, N. Cam, Novel low-cost ultra-wideband, ultra-short-pulse transmitter with MESFET impulse-shaping circuitry for reduced distortion and improved pulse repetition rate. IEEE Microw. Wirel. Compon. Lett. **11**, 208–210 (2001)
3. S. Bourdel, Y. Bachelet, J. Gaubert, R. Vauche, O. Fourquin, N. Dehaese, H. Barthelemy, A 9-pJ/Pulse 1.42-Vpp OOK CMOS UWB pulse generator for the 3.1-10.6 GHz FCC band. IEEE Trans. Microw. Theory Tech. **58**, 65–73 (2010)
4. L. Smaini, C. Tinella, D. Helal, C. Stoecklin, L. Chabert, C. Devaucelle, R. Cattenoz, N. Rinaldi, D. Belot, Single-chip CMOS pulse generator for UWB systems. IEEE J. Solid-State Circuits **41**, 1551–1561 (2006)
5. S. Sanghoon, K. Dong-Wook, H. Songcheol, A CMOS UWB pulse generator for 3-10 GHz applications. IEEE Microw. Wirel. Compon. Lett. **19**, 83–85 (2009)
6. M. R. Yuce, W. Liu, M. S. Chae, J. S. Kim, A wideband telemetry unit for multi-channel neural recording systems. IEEE international conference on ultra-wideband (ICUWB), pp. 612–617, Sept 2007

7. Z. Yunliang, J. D. Zuegel, J. R. Marciante, W. Hui, A 0.18 μm CMOS distributed transversal filter for sub-nanosecond pulse synthesis, in *IEEE Radio and Wireless Symposium*, pp. 563–566, 2006

8. M. Chae, W. Liu, Z. Yang, T. Chen, J. Kim, M. Sivaprakasam, M. Yuce, A 128-channel 6mW wireless neural recording IC with on-the-fly spike sorting and UWB transmitter. IEEE international solid-state circuits conference (ISSCC'08), pp. 146–603, 3–7 Feb 2008

9. Y. Gao, Y. Zheng, S. Diao, W. Toh, C. Ang, M. Je, C. Heng, Low-power ultra-wideband wireless telemetry transceiver for medical sensor applications. IEEE Trans. Biomed. Eng. **58**(3), 768, 772 (2011)

10. Ho Chee Keong, M. R. Yuce, Low data rate ultra wideband ECG monitoring system. IEEE engineering in medicine and biology society conference, pp. 3413–3416, August 2008

11. D.D. Wentzloff, A.P. Chandrakasan, Gaussian pulse generators for subbanded ultra-wideband transmitters. IEEE Trans. Microw. Theory Tech. **54**, 1647–1655 (2006)

12. J. Ryckaert, C. Desset, A. Fort, M. Badaroglu, V. De Heyn, P. Wambacq, G. Van der Plas, S. Donnay, B. Van Poucke, B. Gyselinckx, Ultra-wide-band transmitter for low-power wireless body area networks: design and evaluation. IEEE Trans. Circuits Syst. I Regul. Pap. **52**, 2515–2525 (2005)

13. K. Hyunseok, J. Young Joong, and J. Sungying, Digitally controllable bi-phase CMOS UWB pulse generator. IEEE international conference on ultra-wideband, pp. 442–445, 2005

14. T. Norimatsu, R. Fujiwara, M. Kokubo, M. Miyazaki, A. Maeki, Y. Ogata, S. Kobayashi, N. Koshizuka, K. Sakamura, A UWB-IR transmitter with digitally controlled pulse generator. IEEE J. Solid-State Circuits **42**, 1300–1309 (2007)

15. Z. Ming Jian, L. Bin, W. Zhao Hui, 20-pJ/Pulse 250 Mbps Low-complexity CMOS UWB transmitter for 3–5 GHz applications. IEEE Microw. Wirel. Compon. Lett. **23**, 158–160 (2013)

16. D. Baranauskas, D. Zelenin, A 0.36 W up to 20GS/s DAC for UWB wave formation. IEEE international solid-state circuits conference, pp. 2380–2389, 2006

17. http://www.national.com/pf/DC/ADC12D1800.html#Overview, 2013

18. L. Lampe, K. Witrisal, Challenges and recent advances in IR-UWB system design, in *IEEE International Symposium on Circuits and Systems*, pp. 3288–3291, June 2010

19. D. Barras, R. Meyer-Piening, G. von Bueren, W. Hirt, H. Jaeckel, A low-power baseband ASIC for an energy-collection IR-UWB receiver. IEEE J Solid-State Circuits **44**(6), 1721,1733 (2009)

20. A. Gerosa, S. Soldà, A. Bevilacqua, D. Vogrig, A. Neviani, An energy-detector for noncoherent impulse-radio UWB receivers. IEEE Trans. Circuits Syst. I Regul. Pap. **56**(5), 1030–1040 (2009)

21. L. Jinjin, L. Jianan, S. Zhiyuan, A new transmitted reference based UWB receiver. Int. Conf. Commun. Mobile Comput. **3**, 97–101 (2010)

22. G. F. Tchere, P. Ubolkosold, S. Knedlik, O. Loffeld, Bit error performance of UWB differential transmitted reference systems, in *International Symposium on Communications and Information Technologies*, pp. 609–614, Sep 2006

23. K. Witrisal, G. Leus, G. Janssen, M. Pausini, F. Troesch, T. Zasowski, J. Romme, Noncoherent ultra-wideband systems. IEEE Signal Process. Mag. **26**, 48–66 (2009)

24. L. Zhou, Z. Chen, C. Wang, F. Tzeng, V. Jain, P. Heydari, A 2-Gb/s 130-nm CMOS RF-correlation-based IR-UWB transceiver front-end. IEEE Trans. Microw. Theory Tech. **59**(4), 1117–1130 (2011)

25. C. Geng, Y. Pei, W. Wen, Z. Luan, N. Ge, ASIC implementation of fractionally spaced Rake receiver for high data rate UWB systems. Electron. Lett. **47**(3), 215–217 (2011)

26. W.M. Lovelace, J.K. Townsend, The effects of timing jitter and tracking on the performance of impulse radio. IEEE J. Sel. Areas Commun. **20**, 1646–1651 (2002)

27. O. Mi-Kyung, J. Byunghoo, R. Harjani, P. Dong-Jo, A new noncoherent UWB impulse radio receiver. IEEE Commun. Lett. **9**, 151–153 (2005)

28. A. Idriss, R. Moorfeld, S. Zeisberg, A. Finger, Performance of coherent and non-coherent receivers of UWB communication. Second IFIP international conference on wireless and optical communications networks, pp. 117–122, 6–8 March 2005
29. T. Wei, E. Culurciello, A low-power high-speed ultra-wideband pulse radio transmission system. IEEE Trans. Biomed. Circuits Syst. **3**, 286–292 (2009)
30. J. Colli-Vignarelli, C. Dehollain, A discrete-components impulse-radio ultrawide-band (IR-UWB) transmitter. IEEE Trans. Microw. Theory Tech. **59**, 1141–1146 (2011)
31. M. R. Yuce, K. M. Thotahewa, K. Ho Chee, Development of low-power UWB body sensors, in *International Symposium on Communications and Information Technologies*, pp. 143–148, 2012
32. K. Ho Chee, M. R. Yuce, UWB-WBAN sensor node design. Annual international conference of the IEEE engineering in medicine and biology society, pp. 2176–2179, 2011

Chapter 5
An Ultra-Wideband Sensor Node Development with Dual-Frequency Band for Medical Signal Monitoring

Abstract Impulse Radio-Ultra-wideband (IR-UWB) can be considered as an attractive wireless technology for WBAN applications due to its inherent features, such as low power consuming transmitter design, low complexity hardware implementation, possibility of developing sensor nodes with small form factors and high data rate capability. However, IR-UWB receivers are complex in design and consume large amount of power compared to IR-UWB transmitters. This poses a challenge to use IR-UWB technology in low-power WBAN devices. This chapter discusses the hardware implementation of a dual band communication system for body area network applications that consists of a compact wearable sensor node design and an off-body coordinator node. Hardware architecture of sensor nodes is designed in such a way that it uses UWB for data transmission while a narrow band link is used for data reception. This chapter analyses the design considerations regarding the hardware implementation of compact sensor nodes, such as avoiding the interference between UWB and narrow band sections of the sensor node, Radio Frequency (RF) impedance matching techniques and circuit miniaturization techniques. It also depicts experimental measurements obtained using the dual band communication system.

Keywords IR-UWB · Narrowband · Transmitters · Receivers · ISM · Dual-band · Pulse generators · UWB pulse analysis · UWB spectrum · RF PCB design · Microwave impedance matching

5.1 Introduction

Figure 5.1 shows a commonly used hardware implementation of a sensor node for wireless body area network applications [1]. Sensors are used to sense body signals. Microcontroller handles the digitizing, processing, and formatting of sensor data for wireless transmission. Wireless communication is done via a transceiver that transmits data generated by the micro-controller wirelessly. Together with the

K. M. S. Thotahewa et al., *Ultra Wideband Wireless Body Area Networks*,
DOI: 10.1007/978-3-319-05287-8_5,
© Springer International Publishing Switzerland 2014

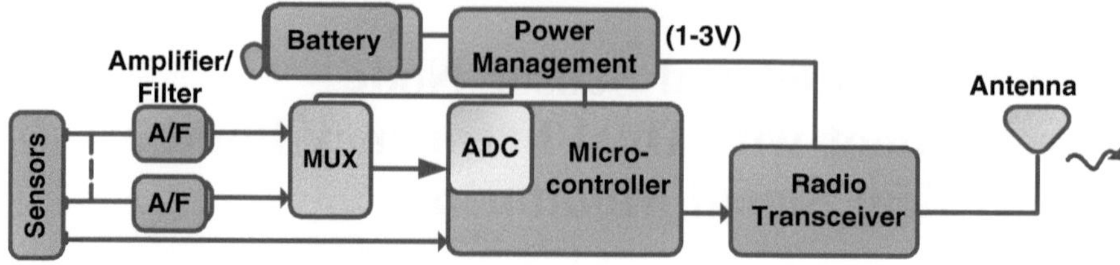

Fig. 5.1 An example of sensor node design for WBAN [1]

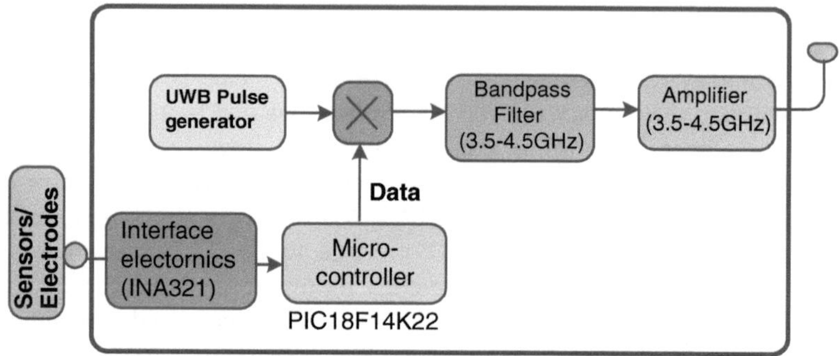

Fig. 5.2 A transmit-only IR-UWB sensor node design [2–4]

antenna, this unit provides the wireless capability for a sensor node. In wireless
sensor network applications, transceiver uses a signal band for both transmitting
data and receiving data. Figure 5.2 shows the block diagram of an IR-UWB sensor
node that does not contain any receiver [2–4]. This design uses a transmit-only
approach to transfer data from sensor nodes to a central coordinator node.

The body area network sensor node presented in this chapter is battery powered
and consists of an IR-UWB transmitter, a 433 MHz Industrial, Scientific and
Medical (ISM) band receiver, an analog interface circuit and a micro-controller
module [5, 6]. The use of an ISM band receiver eradicates the requirement of a
complex UWB receiver at the sensor node, hence greatly reduces the power consumption as well as the design complexity of the sensor node. IR-UWB pulse generator and IR-UWB RF section lies at the core of the sensor node. This chapter
analyses various physical layer properties of IR-UWB signals, such as pulse width,
Pulse Repetition Frequency (PRF), and rise/fall times of pulses in order to design an
IR-UWB pulse generator with a less complex hardware implementation and
enhanced performance. IR-UWB RF section is developed based on an up-conversion
based hardware architecture, where base band pulses are up-converted using a mixer
in order to utilize the higher power contained within the lower half of the frequency
spectrum that belongs to the base band pulse stream generated by the IR-UWB pulse
generator. Hardware design techniques that are followed when integrating a transmitter that operates in UWB frequencies (3.5–4.5 GHz) and a receiver that operates

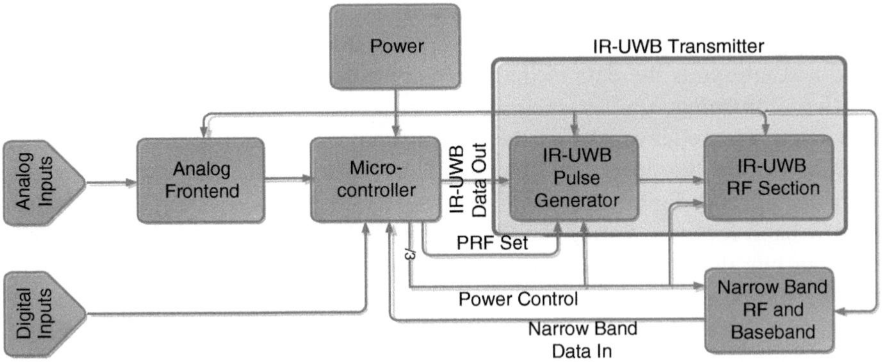

Fig. 5.3 Operational blocks of the dual band sensor node

in 433 MHz ISM band are described in detail herein. This chapter also gives an overview of the control program implemented in the micro-controller in order to achieve efficient operation of the sensor node.

Coordinator node acts as the central controlling device of the Wireless Body Area Network (WBAN) system described in this chapter. It consists of an IR-UWB receiver front-end, a 433 MHz ISM band transmitter, a Field Program-mable Gate Array (FPGA) and a computer that communicates with the FPGA for data gathering purposes. Two different implementations of the IR-UWB receiver front-end are discussed herein. The first generation IR-UWB receiver front-end is made using connectable Radio Frequency (RF) components that are readily available as off-the-shelf RF components. The second-generation IR-UWB receiver front-end circuitry is more compact than the first generation design and is implemented on a four layer PCB. Both these receiver front-end designs are intended to operate off-the body and receive data from on-body dual band sensor nodes; hence can be powered using a commercial power supply.

5.2 Dual Band Sensor Node Design: Employing a Narrow-Band Receiver in the Sensor Node

The basic block diagram of the proposed dual band sensor node is shown in Fig. 5.3. It consists of five major operational blocks that are mentioned below.

- *IR-UWB pulse generator:*
This unit generates narrow IR-UWB pulses, and combines them with the data bits produced by the micro-controller.
- *IR-UWB RF section:*
It filters and up-converts the base band IR-UWB pulses into the target frequency range of 3.5–4.5 GHz.

- ***Narrow band RF and base band section:***
It is designed to communicate with the coordinator node using the 433 MHz ISM band and interprets the data to the micro-controller.
- ***Micro-controller:***
The micro-controller works as the central controlling unit that coordinates the operation of all the operational blocks of the sensor node. This includes reading both analog and digital data from the respective inputs, reading data from the narrow band receiver, setting the PRF of the IR-UWB pulse generator, generating the data bits that should be transmitted using the IR-UWB transmitter and controlling the power to various sections of the sensor node in order to enable the sleep mode operation. In addition, micro-controller handles all the functions related to the operation of Medium Access Control (MAC) protocol at the sensor node.
- ***Analog front-end:***
This section interfaces the analog input signals, such as Electrocardiography (ECG) with the Analog to Digital Converter (ADC) of the micro-controller.
- ***Power management unit:***
The responsibility of the power management unit is to supply and control power to all operational parts of the circuit. All the RF related circuits of the sensor nodes, such as IR-UWB transmitter components and narrow band receiver module are powered with a 3 V supply while rest of the hardware uses a 3.3 V power supply.

Each of these main operational blocks of the dual band sensor node are described in detail in the following sub sections.

5.2.1 Pulse Generation Techniques

IR-UWB pulse generator lies at the core of the IR-UWB transmitter. An up-conversion pulse generation technique is utilized in this design considering the advantages offered by this technique that are discussed in Chap. 4. The up-conversion pulse generation technique uses a mixer to up-convert the base band pulses generated by a pulse generator, and filters the up-converted pulses so that the pulse spectrum falls within the intended bandwidth (3.5–4.5 GHz for the sensor node described in this chapter) before transmission. This technique offers the highest power efficiency for a UWB transmitter developed using off-the-shelf components.

In the sensor node design described in this chapter, IR-UWB pulses are generated by passing a periodic square wave signal and its time-delayed version through a XOR gate as shown in Fig. 5.4. Two sets of buffers with different supply voltages are used to introduce different delay levels to the signal [7, 8]. The work presented in [9] shows that the delay between the input and the output of a buffer depends on the applied supply voltage to the buffer. This relationship is given by (5.1):

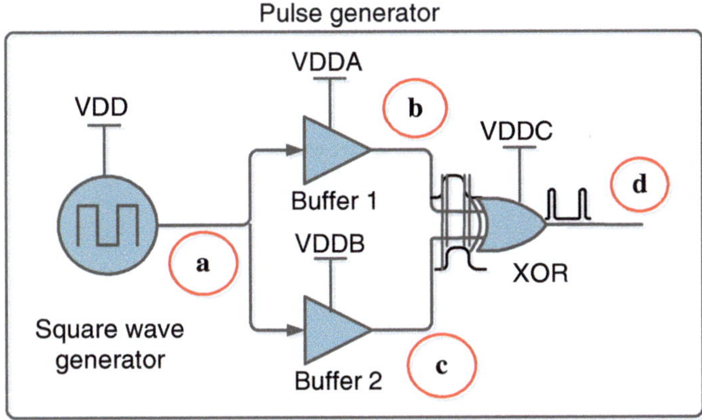

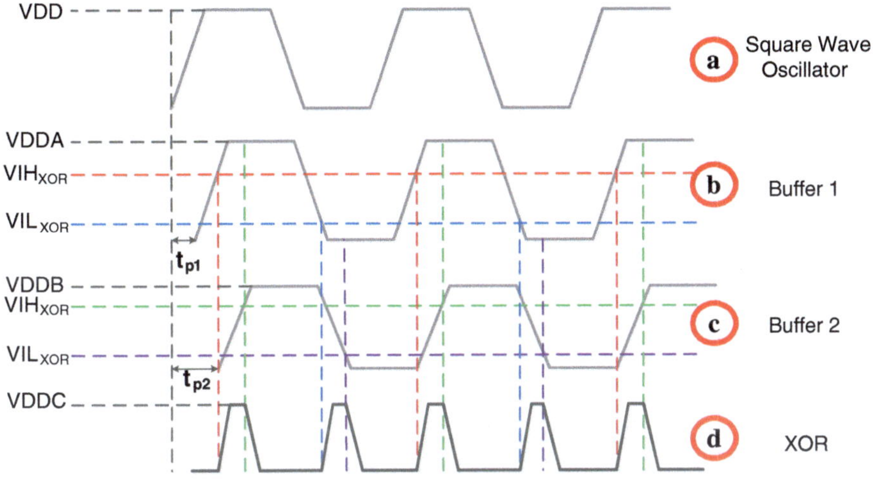

VIH$_{XOR}$ – Input high voltage of the XOR gate

VIL$_{XOR}$ – Input low voltage of the XOR gate

t_{p1} – Propagation delay of the Buffer 1

t_{p2} – Propagation delay of the Buffer 2

Fig. 5.4 IR-UWB pulse generation **a** output of the square wave generator **b**, **c** output from buffer 1 and 2 **d** narrow pulse stream after the XOR gate

$$t_p = \frac{C_L}{2V_{DD}}\left(\frac{1}{k_1}+\frac{1}{k_2}\right) \tag{5.1}$$

where t_p is the propagation delay caused by the buffer, C_L is the load capacitance, V_{DD} is the supply voltage of the buffer, and k_1, k_2 are the gain factors. By passing identical versions of a square wave signal through two identical buffers, it is possible to keep C_L, k_1 and k_2 common to both buffers; hence the output delay generated by each buffer can be solely controlled by adjusting the V_{DD} of each buffer. The adjustable voltage range of the buffers depends on the input high voltage specifications of buffers and XOR gate. The condition that should be satisfied by supply voltages of the buffers in order to generate a narrow pulse stream can be shown as:

$$\frac{VDDA}{\beta} \geq VDDB \geq VIH_{XOR}, \ where \ \beta = \frac{VIH_{Buffer}}{VDDB} \tag{5.2}$$

where $VDDA$ and $VDDB$ are supply voltages of the two buffers, VIH_{XOR} is the input high voltage of the XOR gate, and VIH_{Buffer} is the input high voltage of the buffer.

The square wave input to the two delay lines is generated using a square wave oscillator. In reality, the output of a square wave oscillator forms a trapezoidal signal due to the finite output capacitance at the square wave output. As shown in Fig. 5.4, this results in a narrow trapezoidal pulse stream at the output of the XOR gate.

With the correct amount of delay setting in the buffers, it is possible to bring the rising and falling edges of these trapezoidal waveforms close together, forming an approximated triangular pulse waveform at the output of the XOR gate. The power spectrum of the triangular pulses has suppressed side lobes compared to that of the rectangular pulses [9]. Hence, the power loss that might occur by using a square wave pulse as the base band pulse for UWB RF section can be reduced by using the triangular shaped pulses generated using this technique. The IR-UWB pulses generated by this mechanism are then up- converted using a mixer and sent through a Band Pass Filter (BPF) for the purpose of spectral shaping. This is done in the IR-UWB RF section, which is discussed in a subsequent section. The properties of the IR-UWB pulses, such as rise time, pulse width and PRF play an important role in the output of the IR-UWB pulse generator. It is important to analyze these properties in order to parameterize the circuit components of the IR-UWB pulse generator.

5.2.2 Analysis of UWB Pulse Properties

This section analyses the properties of IR-UWB pulses, such as pules width, rise time and PRF, in order to investigate their effects on transmit spectrum of the UWB signals.

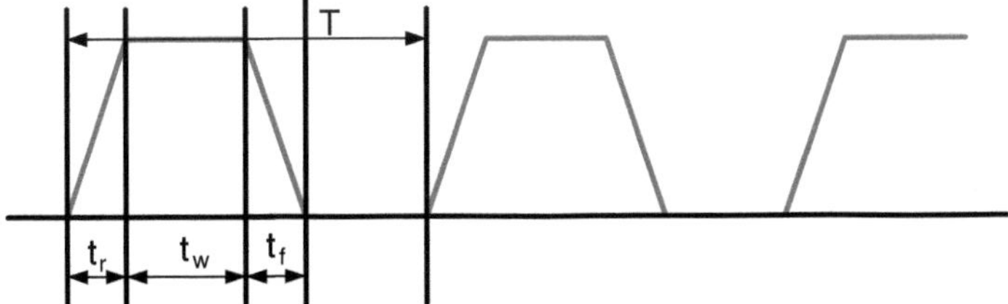

Fig. 5.5 Trapezoidal pulse train

5.2.2.1 Effect of Pulse Width on UWB Transmit Spectrum

The trapezoidal waveform generated by the pulse generator can be characterised by properties, such as rise and fall times (t_r, t_f), pulse width (t_w) and pulse period (T), as shown in Fig. 5.5.

If equal rise and fall times are assumed for UWB pulses (*i.e.* $t_r = t_f$), the basic UWB pulse ($p(t)$) can be expressed in following manner:

$$p(t) = \begin{cases} 0 & t < -t_r - t_w/2 \\ A(t + t_r + t_w/2)/t_r & -t_r - t_w/2 \le t \le -t_r/2 \\ A & -t_w/2 < t < t_w/2 \\ A(t_r + t_w/2 - t)/t_r & t_w/2 \le t \le t_w/2 + t_r \\ 0 & t > t_w/2 + t_r \end{cases} \tag{5.3}$$

where A is the maximum pulse amplitude, t_r is the rise and fall times of the pulse and t_w is the pulse width. The Fourier series expansion of the pulse train can be expressed as below:

$$x(t) = \frac{2A(t_w + t_r)}{T} \sum_{n=n1}^{n2} \frac{\sin \pi f_n t_r}{\pi f_n t_r} \frac{\sin \pi f_n (t_w + t_r)}{\pi f_n (t_w + t_r)} \cos(2\pi n f t) \tag{5.4}$$

where $f_n = n/T$, T is the time period of the pulse train, and n is an integer, $n_1 = f_1/f$ and $n_2 = f_2/f$ where f_1 and f_2 are upper and lower cut off frequencies for the BPF. The sensor nodes described in this chapter are intended to operate in the frequency range of 3.5–4.5 GHz. Hence $f_1 = 3.5$ GHz and $f_2 = 4.5$ GHz for this particular design. This frequency band is chosen in order to avoid possible interference that can be generated due to the operation of other equipment in RF bands, such as 5 GHz WLAN. The first *sinc* function in (5.4) is determined by the rise time of the pulses, while the second *sinc* function depends on both rise time and pulse width. This results in an output waveform that is a function of both rise time and pulse width.

Transmit spectrums of simulated UWB pulse streams with pulse widths of 1, 0.5 and 2 ns are shown in Fig. 5.6. These UWB transmit spectrums are obtained using simulations conducted in Advanced Design Systems, which is a commercial

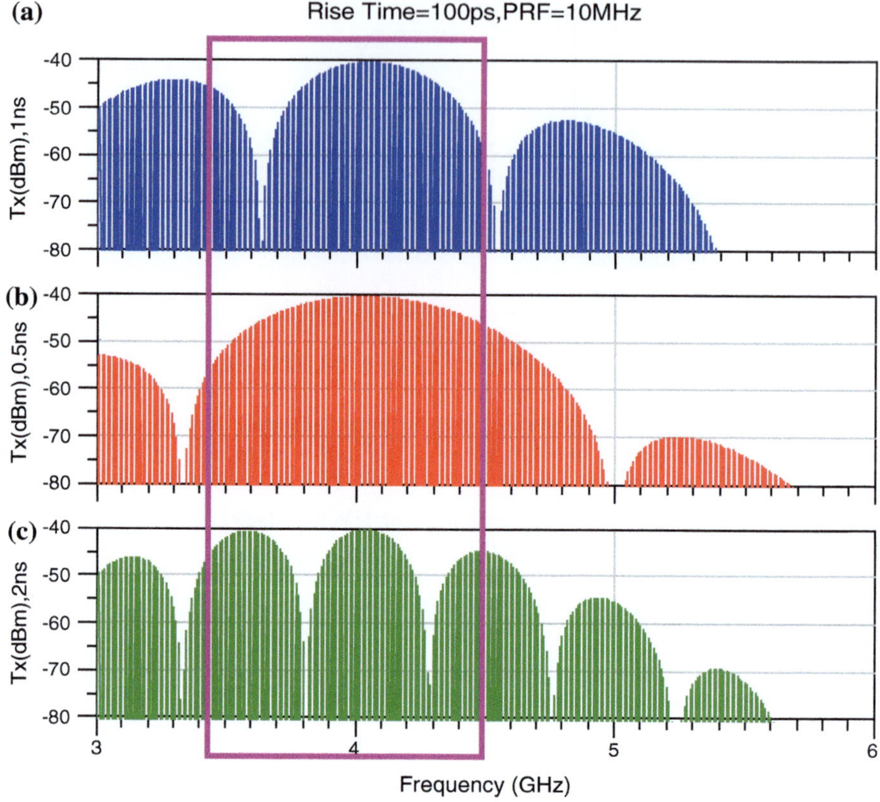

Fig. 5.6 Transmit spectrum for **a** 1 ns pulse width **b** 0.5 ns pulse width **c** 2 ns pulse width

RF simulation software. Simulations use the same pulse generation technique as described in Sect. 5.2.1. Rise and fall times of the pulses are set to be 100 ps and a PRF of 10 MHz is used for the simulated pulse train. In an IR-UWB system, UWB pulse width is responsible for the bandwidth of a single *sinc* component of the spectrum. It also determines the number of nulls that occur within the band of interest, which is a 1 GHz bandwidth centered at 4 GHz in these simulations (this is highlighted by the framed areas in the figures). Occurrence of nulls within the band of interest affects the transmitted signal adversely. As can be seen from the respective time domain signals for each case in Fig. 5.7, occurrence of nulls tends to reduce the pulse amplitude of the time domain pulse. It also results in creating two adjacent time domain pulses instead of a single pulse, which makes the pulse reception more complicated. Hence, it is preferable to use a pulse width, which does not create any nulls within the band of interest. It can be determined form (5.4) that a null in the spectrum occurs at every integer multiple of $\frac{1}{t_r+t_w}$.

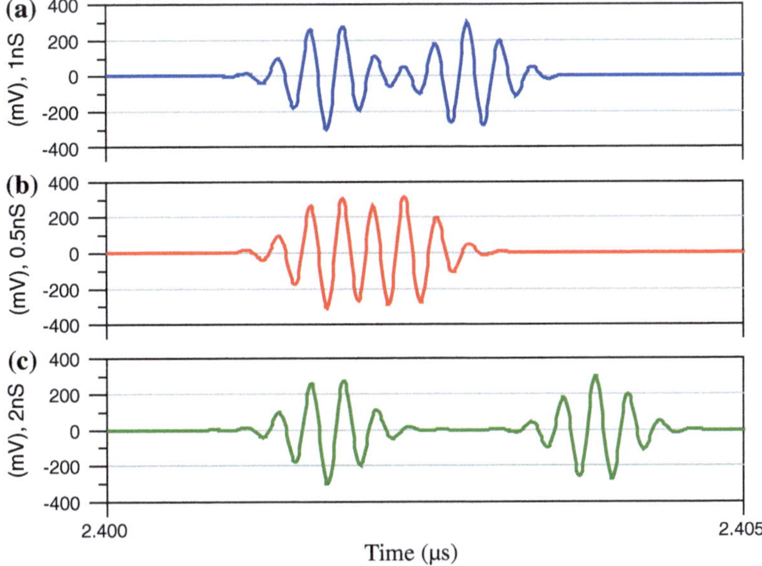

Fig. 5.7 Transmit pulse for **a** 1 ns pulse width **b** 0.5 ns pulse width **c** 2 ns pulse width

5.2.2.2 Effect of Rise Time on UWB Transmit Spectrum

Transmit spectrums for IR-UWB pulse trains with 100 and 250 ps rise times are shown in Fig. 5.8. A pulse width of 0.5 ns and a PRF of 10 MHz are used in all pulse streams for the purpose of comparison between signals. By comparison of the output power spectrums shown in Fig. 5.8, it can be seen that the position of nulls within the transmit spectrum depends on the rise time of IR-UWB pulses. In fact, it can be observed that the occurrence of a null in the transmit spectrum of UWB signals depends on both rise time and pulse width, while the bandwidth of a single *sinc* component of the spectrum depends only on the pulse width. Occurrence of a null at the center frequency causes the time domain amplitude to be lower, causing weaker transmitted signal strength as shown in Fig. 5.9. It is preferable for the peak of the transmit spectrum to be aligned with the center frequency of the intended band of interest in order to obtain the maximum signal amplitude. The condition that should be satisfied in order to obtain a spectral peak at the intended center frequency can be derived as:

$$f_c.(t_r + t_w) = 0.5\gamma \tag{5.5}$$

where f_c is the centre frequency and γ is an odd integer. In an up-conversion IR-UWB transmitter, such as the one discussed in this chapter, the base band portion of the UWB pulse spectrum (*i.e.* the low frequency portion) is selected using a filter and is then up-converted to the frequency range of interest using a

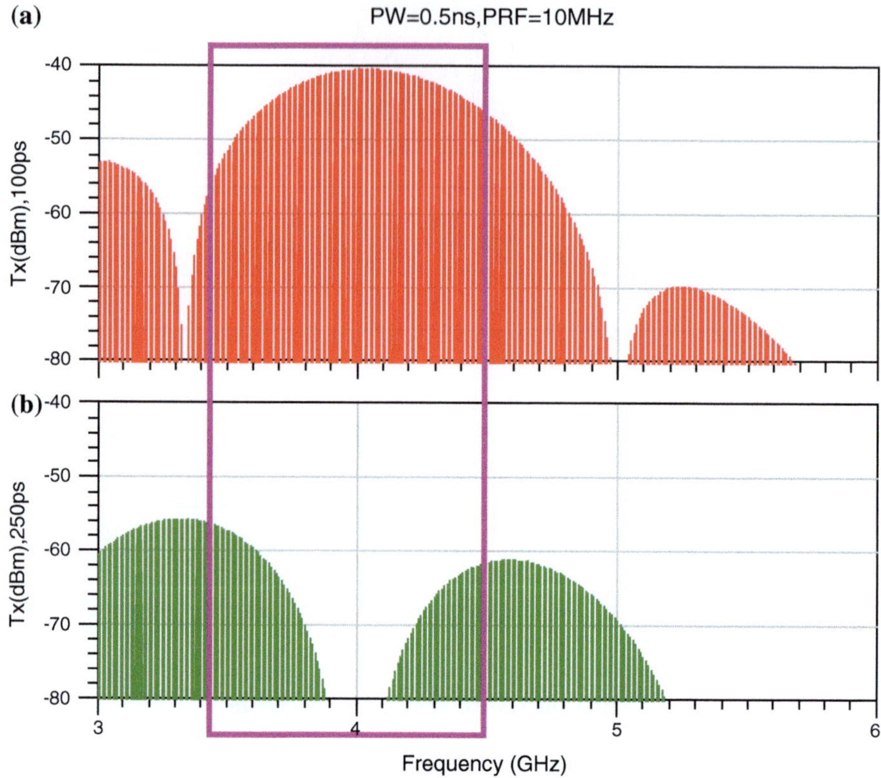

Fig. 5.8 Transmit spectrum for **a** 100 ps rise time **b** 250 ps rise time

mixer. For example, the UWB RF section discussed in this chapter filters out the lower frequency portion within the frequency band of 0–1.4 GHz from the base band pulse spectrum, and up-converts it by 4 GHz using a mixer. Hence, the occurrence of nulls in the band of interest can be avoided as long as the bandwidth of the first *sinc* component that belongs to the base band portion of the spectrum is sufficiently large to cover the base band bandwidth of interest (0–1.4 GHz for this design). In other words, only the pulse width plays a significant role in characterizing the transmit spectrum in an up-conversion transmitter. Although it is possible to control the pulse width by controlling the supply voltages of the buffer amplifiers, the rise time of the square pulses depends on the electrical characteristics of the components, such as the square wave generator and the XOR gate, and is hard to control. Hence, by using the up-conversion technique as suggested in this chapter, it is possible to avoid the requirement to control the rise time of the pulses in order to generate a UWB pulse stream with a spectrum that has no nulls in the band of interest. The up-conversion technique suggested in this chapter only depends on the easily controllable pulse width for the latter purpose.

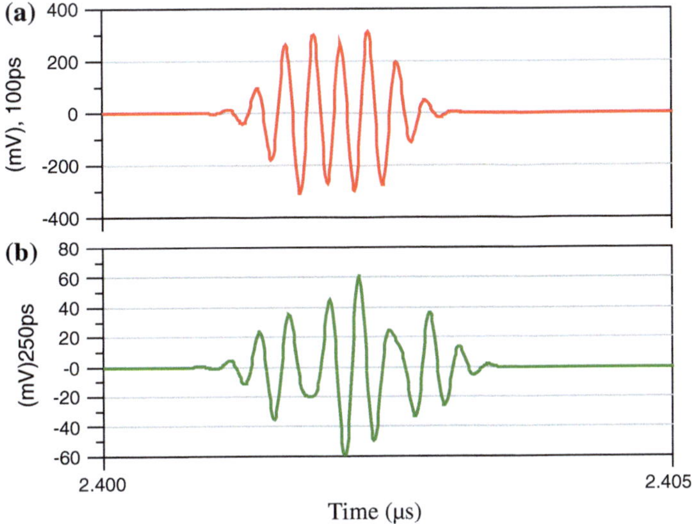

Fig. 5.9 Transmit pulse for **a** 100 ps rise time **b** 250 ps rise time

5.2.2.3 Optimization of PRF for UWB Transmit Spectrum

As depicted in Fig. 5.10, PRF affects the number of spectral lines and their amplitudes that lie within a certain bandwidth. A higher PRF system tends to create lesser number of spectral lines that are higher in amplitude, while a lower PRF results in spectral lines that are closer to each other with lower amplitudes. As a result, the peak transmit power for higher PRF systems will be comparatively higher than that of lower PRF systems. These spectral lines can be characterised by the PSD of the IR-UWB signal, which consists of a continuous spectrum and a line spectrum [9]. The continuous spectrum is determined by pulse width and rise time of the IR-UWB pulse stream while the line spectrum corresponds to the PRF. The amplitude of the line spectrum tends to be *10.log (PRF/1 MHz)* higher than the continuous spectrum, for a resolution bandwidth of 1 MHz selected according to the FCC regulations [9]. They appear at *1/T* Hz apart from each other, where *1/T = PRF*. These spectral lines create overshoots above the FCC spectral mask. Even after averaging over a 1 MHz bandwidth, they result in higher average powers, which will violate the FCC regulations. For an application that requires a high PRF, these spectral lines can be reduced by using a modulation scheme that makes the transmitted signal equiprobable [9]. Similarly, using a duty cycled IR-UWB data transmission will reduce the spectral overshoots of a high PRF IR-UWB system.

The amplitude of IR-UWB pulses does not determine the spectral shape or locations of the nulls, rather it determines the peak amplitude of the transmit spectrum. The amplitude of the IR-UWB pulses can be varied in order to contain the transmit spectrum within the FCC spectral mask.

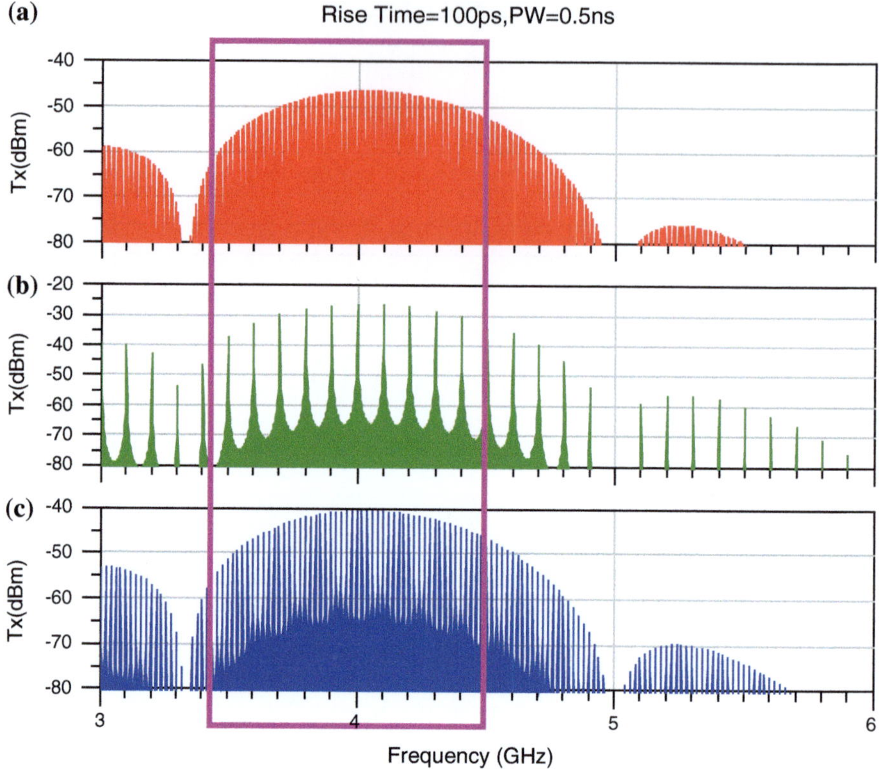

Fig. 5.10 Transmit spectrums for PRF s **a** 10 MHz **b** 100 MHz **c** 50 MHz

5.2.3 *Implementation of the Pulse Generator*

A reconfigurable square wave oscillator is used as the source for the pulse generator circuit. *LTC6905* programmable oscillator by Linear Technology is chosen for this purpose mainly due to its short rise and fall times [10]. This is a resistor set oscillator, in which the oscillation frequency (f_{osc}) can be varied by changing the external resistance value (R_{SET}) of the oscillator calibration input using a single resistor according to the following equation [10]:

$$f_{osc} = \left(\frac{168.5\,MHz \times 10\,k\Omega}{R_{SET}} + 1.5\,MHz \right) \times \frac{1}{N}, N = \left\{ \begin{array}{l} 1, DIV\,pin = V^+ \\ 2, DIV\,pin = OPEN \\ 4, DIV\,pin = GND \end{array} \right\}$$

$$(5.6)$$

In an attempt to change the oscillation frequency without manual intervention, *AD5286* programmable resistor from Analog Devices [11] is used to set the

Fig. 5.11 Layout of the reconfigurable square wave generator

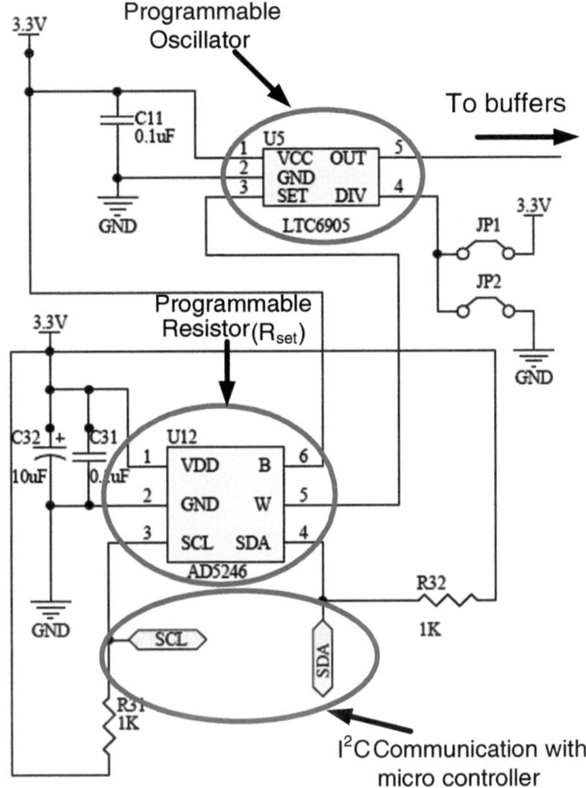

Table 5.1 Main components of the IR-UWB pulse generator

Functional block	Component	Manufacturer
Square wave oscillator	LTC6905	Linear technology [10]
Programmable resistor	AD5286	Analog devices [11]
Buffer	NC7WZ126	Fairchild semiconductor [12]
XOR gate	NC7SZ86	Fairchild semiconductor [12]

resistance value of the oscillator calibration input. It is possible to change the resistance of this programmable resistor through Inter-Integrated Circuit (I^2C) communication with a micro-controller, enabling reconfigurations of the PRF without intervening with the circuitry. Circuit diagram for this configuration is shown in Fig. 5.11. Set of components used in the implementation of the pulse generator is shown in Table 5.1.

Circuit components for buffers and XOR gate are chosen considering their fast transition times and small form factors. Two transmission line sections between square wave oscillator and buffers, and between buffers and XOR gate are designed such that the delay introduced by the signal propagation through each path is

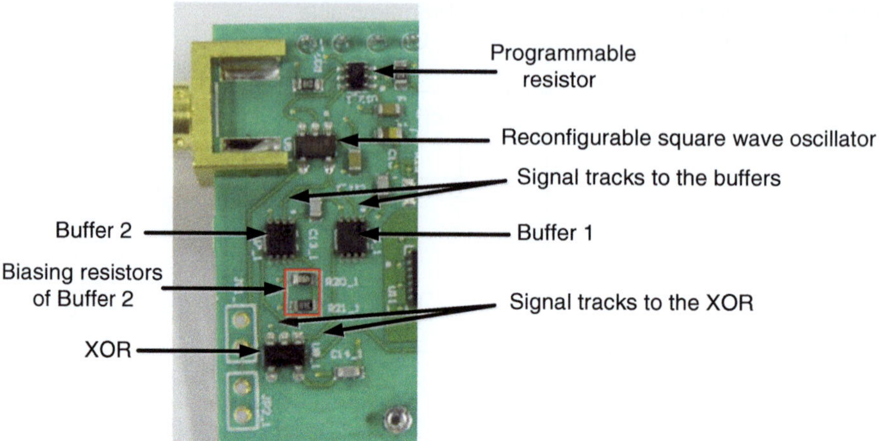

Fig. 5.12 PCB implementation of the pulse generator

identical. This is necessary to make sure that the delay in each signal propagation path is only affected by the voltage-controlled delay introduced by the buffers. The propagation delay for the transmission lines are calculated using (5.7) [13].

$$t_p = \frac{B_r \cdot \sqrt{\varepsilon_r}}{300} \left(\frac{\text{ns}}{\text{mm}} \right),$$

$$B_r = 0.8566 + 0.0294 \cdot \ln(w) + 0.00239\,h + 0.0101\varepsilon_r \tag{5.7}$$

where ε_r is the dielectric constant of the PCB substrate, w is the width of the transmission line in *mils* and h is the height from the nearest ground plane to the transmission line in *mils*. The pulse generator implemented on the sensor node PCB is shown in Fig. 5.12.

The relationship between signal bandwidth, pulse width and center frequency for an IR-UWB pulse stream generated using the up-conversion method is given by (5.8) [14].

$$B \cdot t_w = 2 \cdot (1 - \beta) \cdot \alpha \tag{5.8}$$

where B is the signal bandwidth, t_w is the pulse width and α and β are dimensionless scalar values given by:

$$\beta = 1 - \frac{B}{2f_c} \tag{5.9}$$

$$\frac{sinc(\pi \cdot (1 + \beta) \cdot \alpha) - sinc(\pi \cdot (1 - \beta) \cdot \alpha)}{sinc(2\pi \cdot \alpha) - 1} = 0.3162 \tag{5.10}$$

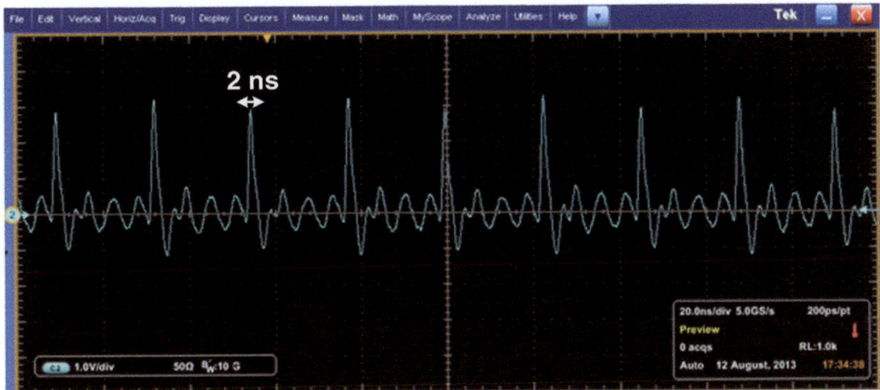

Fig. 5.13 The base band pulse stream generated by the IR-UWB pulse generator

These equations determine the maximum pulse width that the pulse generator should generate in order to cover a certain signal bandwidth around a particular center frequency. By solving these equations it can be estimated that a pulse width of 2 ns will give a transmit spectrum that will cover the intended transmission frequency range of 3.5–4.5 GHz with the center frequency at 4 GHz. A pulse width of 2 ns can be achieved in the pulse generator shown in Fig. 5.12 by choosing the supply voltages of the two buffers to be 3.3 V and 3 V. The supply voltage of the XOR gate determines the peak amplitude of the IR-UWB pulse stream. The base band pulse stream generated by the pulse generator at a 40 MHz PRF is shown in Fig. 5.13.

5.2.4 IR-UWB RF Section

IR-UWB RF section is responsible for the up-conversion of the base band IR-UWB pulse stream into the intended frequency range of 3.5–4.5 GHz. Basic block diagram of the IR-UWB RF section used in this sensor node design is shown in Fig. 5.14.

The data generated by the micro-controller is modulated by the IR-UWB pulse stream using an AND gate before entering the RF portion of the circuit. The base band pulse stream produced by the UWB pulse generator consists of a power spectrum with several frequency lobes (*sinc* components) spread throughout the UWB bandwidth. Amplitudes of these frequency lobes decrease towards the upper part of the UWB spectrum as shown in Fig. 5.15a. UWB RF section employs a Low Pass Filter (LPF) in order to filter out the 0–1.4 GHz section of the UWB pulse spectrum. This portion of the spectrum is of the highest power compared to rest of the spectrum. Filtered spectrum is then shifted using a mixer and a Voltage Controlled Oscillator (VCO) operating at 4 GHz. A band pass filter is used at the

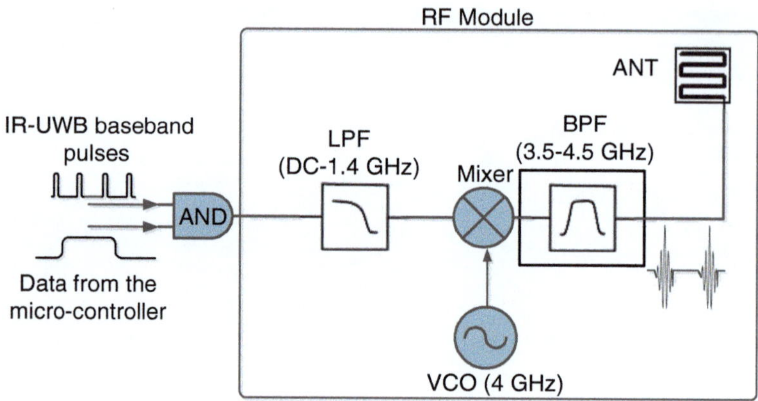

Fig. 5.14 The block diagram of the IR-UWB RF section

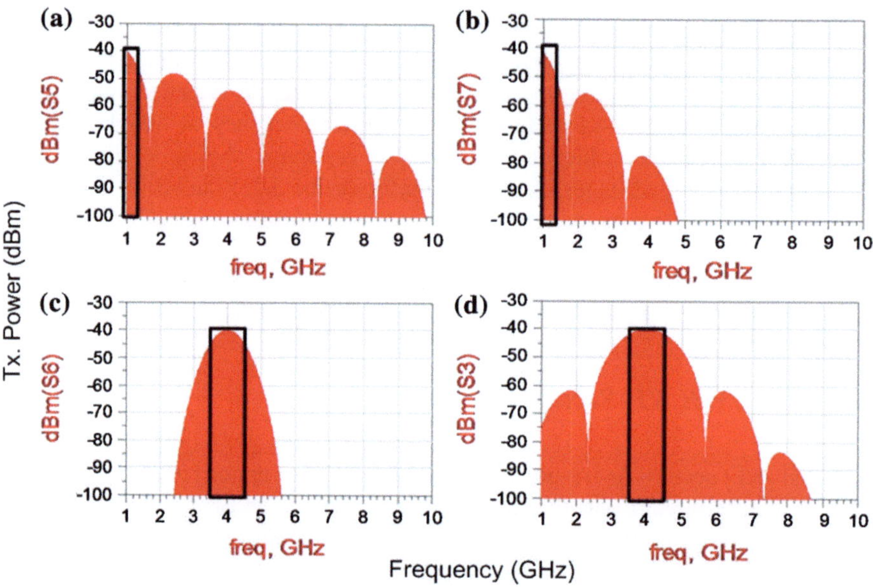

Fig. 5.15 Frequency spectrum of VCO based sensor node at **a** UWB pulse generator output **b** 1.4 GHz LPF output **c** mixer output **d** 3.5–4.5 GHz BPF output

output of the mixer in order to contain the UWB signals within the 3.5–4.5 GHz band.

Figure 5.16 depicts the hardware implementation of the UWB RF section on the sensor node PCB. Co-planar wave-guide transmission lines with 50 Ω impedance matching are used for all the RF tracks of the circuit. Table 5.2 shows major components used in the design of the IR-UWB RF section. The VCO is

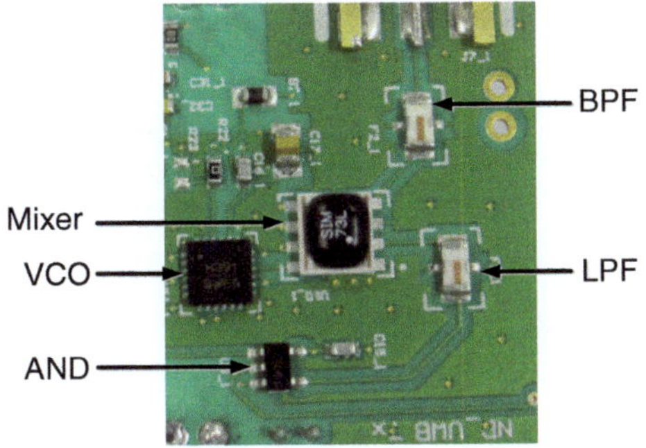

Fig. 5.16 Hardware implementation of the IR-UWB RF section

Table 5.2 Main components of the IR-UWB RF section

Functional block	Component	Manufacturer
Mixer	SIM-73L+	Mini circuits [15]
BPF	BFCN-4440+	Mini circuits [15]
LPF	LFCN-1400+	Mini circuits [15]
VCO	HMC391LP4	Hittite microwave [16]
AND gate	NC7SZ08M5	Fairchild semiconductor [12]

tuned to operate at 4 GHz, which is used as the center frequency for the UWB RF transmission. It can operate at a peak output power of 7 dBm while consuming a peak current of 30 mA. However, it is biased to operate at one third of its output power in order to reduce the power consumption of the design. The mixer can operate at a conversion loss of 6.2 dBm under these operating conditions.

This method of pulse generation has a distinct advantage in terms of power consumption over the direct conversion UWB pulse generation technique, where the lower amplitude frequency lobe within the 3.5–4.5 GHz band is directly filtered out and amplified in order to transmit at a spectral amplitude closer to the FCC spectral mask. It can be observed that the up-conversion UWB transmitter can generate a pulse stream at a close spectral amplitude to the FCC spectral mask without using an amplifier. Hence, this method offers an energy efficient solution for IR-UWB transmission. The time domain RF IR-UWB pulses emitted by the transmitter at a 40 MHz PRF is depicted in Fig. 5.17 together with its transmit frequency spectrum in Fig. 5.18.

5.2.5 The 433 MHz ISM Band Receiver

The receiver in the sensor node is a narrow band receiver that operates in the 433 MHz *ISM* band. *RX5500* ISM band amplifier sequenced hybrid receiver chip by RFM [17], which is an off-the-shelf narrow band receiver chip, is chosen due to its low operating power, high electromagnetic interference rejection and small size. It can operate using both On-Off Keying (OOK) and Amplitude Shift Keying

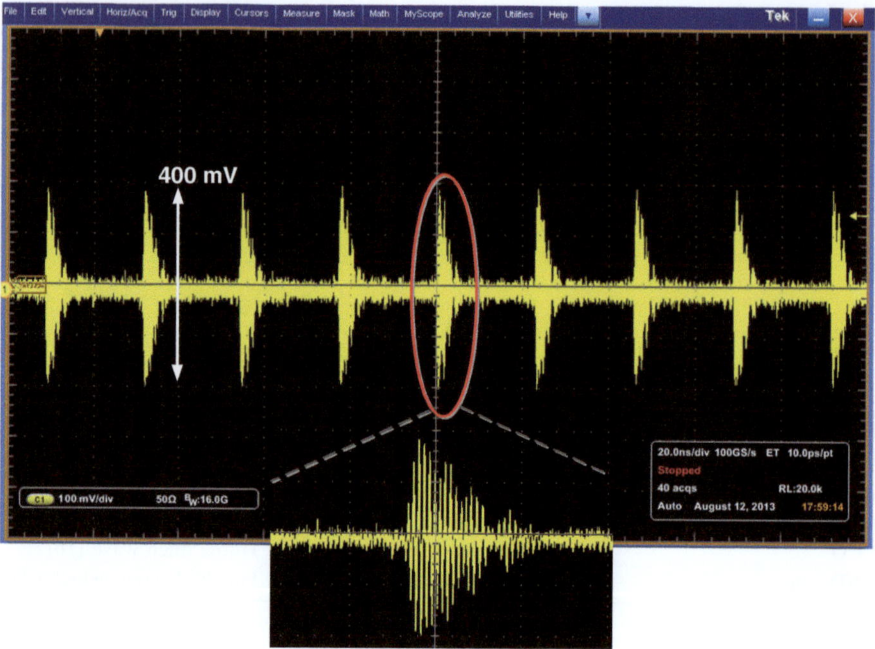

Fig. 5.17 Time domain IR-UWB pulses emitted by the IR-UWB transmitter

(ASK) modulation methods. It operates in low current mode around a power consumption of 5 mW even under the continuous operation. The power overhead introduced by this addition is much lower than using an IR-UWB receiver at the sensor node end. In this manner, it is possible for the coordinator node of the network to send control commands to the sensor node, allowing several sensor nodes to operate in a coordinated network. An impedance matching circuit made out of inductors and capacitors is used in order to match the impedance between the antenna side and the receiver side of the circuit. Narrow band receiver converts the received ISM band RF signal into a base band bit stream that can be read by the micro-controller.

5.2.6 Micro-controller

Micro-controller acts as the central controlling module of the sensor node. It is also responsible for the operation of the MAC protocol at the sensor node. *PIC18F14K22* micro-controller is used in the sensor design because of its low power consumption and the ability to operate with very few external components [18]. The micro-controller is able to control the power given to the base band and RF portions of the sensor node. Hence, it can shut down the RF and base band

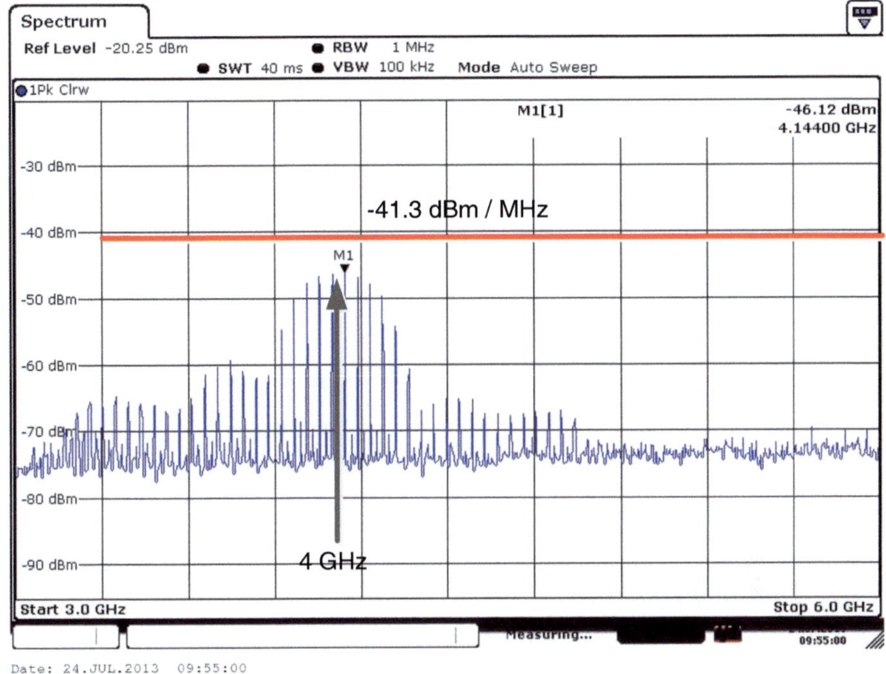

Fig. 5.18 Transmit spectrum at 40 MHz PRF

sections during an intermittent data transmission situation to reduce the power consumption of the sensor node. The micro-controller also acts as the mediator for analog and digital data inputs. It performs the analog to digital conversion using a ten-bit ADC, determines the transmission format and the modulation scheme, and sets the data rate.

The ADC of the sensor node can operate at 20 kHz sampling rate, which is sufficient for physiological signals, such as ECG. The ADC can operate during the sleep mode without consuming much power, hence sensor data acquisition can be performed in between the data transmission periods. The micro-controller runs an internal clock that can operate at a maximum frequency of 60 MHz. IR-UWB pulse rate is independent of the data rate and is arranged by the pulse generator. The UWB pulses generated by the pulse generator are multiplied with the binary data bits created by the micro-controller using an AND gate. The micro-controller used in this design can generate data up to a data rate of 5 Mbps using its digital output pins. Hence, the maximum data rate that can be generated by a sensor node is limited to 5 Mbps. It should be noted that higher data rates could be achieved by choosing a micro-controller with higher performance at the cost of slightly higher power consumption. The implementation of the MAC protocol in the micro-controller is discussed further in Chap. 6.

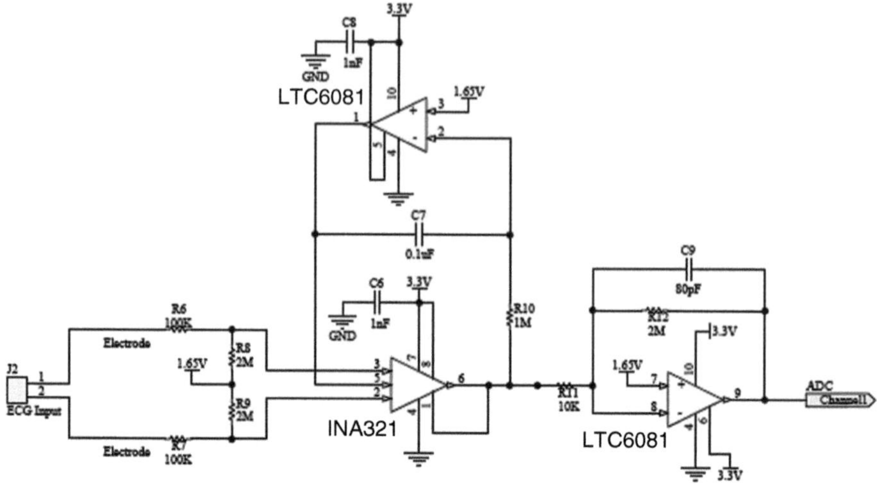

Fig. 5.19 Analog front-end of the sensor node

5.2.7 Analog Front-End

The analog front-end of the sensor node is designed to amplify low voltage
physiological signals, such as ECG. ECG signals generate a waveform with peak
amplitude of approximately 500 μV and a frequency of 100 Hz. During the first
stage of the front-end, low voltage, analog input signals are amplified by 14 dB
using the *INA321* instrumentation amplifier [19]. The second stage of the front-end
acts as an active LPF with a cut-off frequency of 100 Hz and a gain of 46 dB. This
is implemented using *LTC6081* precision dual output amplifier [10]. These components are selected for the analog front-end mainly due to their high common
mode rejection ratio. The schematic of the analog front-end is depicted in
Fig. 5.19.

5.2.8 Power Supply Management

The LP5996 dual linear regulator [19] regulates the power to the sensor node. RF
portions of the circuit are powered using a 3 V regulated power line while rest of
the circuit is powered using a 3.3 V supply. Power to each individual section of the
circuit can be independently controlled by the micro-controller, leading way to
power efficient operation of the sensor node. All the power supply pins of the
sensor node are connected to the power plane of the PCB using vias.

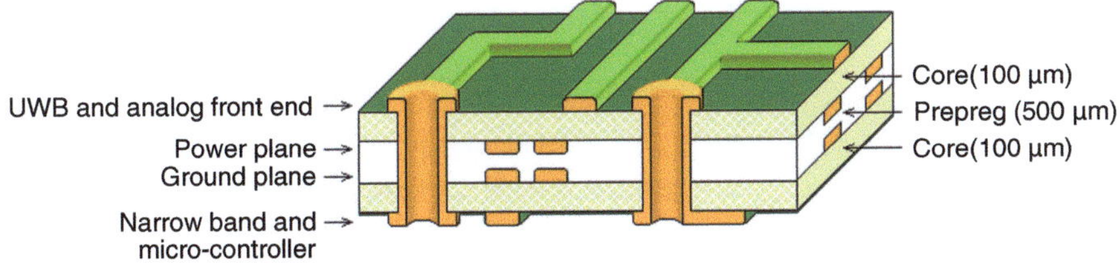

Fig. 5.20 Layer stack up of the sensor node PCB

5.2.9 Sensor Node Integration and Design Considerations

The sensor node is implemented on a four layer PCB in order to preserve the compactness of the sensor design while minimising the electromagnetic interference that occur due to the simultaneous operation of the narrow band and UWB RF sections. RO4350 by Rogers is chosen as the PCB core material due to its low dielectric losses at the frequencies of interest and immunity against cross talk and noise.

Interference mitigation is a major concern for the dual band sensor node design. This design employs two techniques in order to minimise the possible interference between the narrow band and UWB sections of the circuit. The first strategy is to design a regionalised circuit structure using a four-layer PCB design as shown in Fig. 5.20. The use of power and ground planes in between the RF signal layers improves the immunity against cross talk, and improves the noise performance of the circuit by as much as 15 dB [20].

Use of separate ground layers for UWB and narrow band sections is employed as the second technique to minimise interference between the two RF sections. These ground layers are connected in a single spot using a ferrite bead that prevents the exchange of high frequency noise between the two RF sections of the sensor node. Power supplies to all the components are decoupled using bypass capacitors. A ferrite bead is added in series with the power supply of the narrow band receiver in order to prevent the high frequency noise that might leak to the power plane from the UWB transmitter. Many grounded vias are used near all the RF components, such as VCO and mixer, in order to prevent the occurrence of current loops that degrade the signal quality. Stacked micro vias are used for multilayer routing of RF and data signals in order to improve the immunity against Electromagnetic Interference (EMI) [21].

All RF signals are routed using Co-Planar Wave Guides (CPWG) with impedance matched to 50 Ω. The use of CPWG is preferred to route RF transmission lines over the micro-strip lines due to the lower loss tangent and the possibility of narrowing the RF traces in order to match the component pad dimensions. The impedance of the RF tracks is obtained using (5.11) [22].

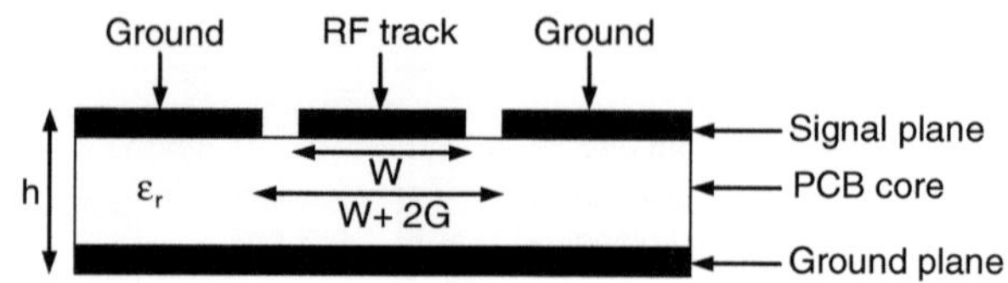

Fig. 5.21 CPWG parameters

$$Z_0 = \frac{60\pi}{\varepsilon_{eff}} \frac{1}{\frac{K(k)}{K(k')} + \frac{K(k_1)}{K(k_1')}} \text{ ohms},$$

$$k = \frac{W}{W + 2G}, \quad k' = \sqrt{1 - k^2},$$

$$k_1 = \frac{\tanh\left(\frac{\pi W}{4h}\right)}{\tanh\left(\frac{\pi(W+2G)}{4h}\right)}, \qquad k_1' = \sqrt{1 - k_1^2},$$

$$\varepsilon_{eff} = \frac{1 + \varepsilon_r \frac{K(k')K(k_1)}{K(k)K(k_1')}}{1 + \frac{K(k')K(k_1)}{K(k)K(k_1')}}, \quad K(k) = \int_0^1 \frac{dt}{\sqrt{(1 - t^2)(1 - k^2 t^2)}} \qquad (5.11)$$

where Z_0 is the impedance of the CPWG, ε_r is the relative permittivity of the PCB material, W, G, and h are CPWG parameters as depicted in Fig. 5.21.

A block diagram showing the overall integration of the sensor node is depicted in Fig. 5.22. The time domain signals obtained at various places of the sensor node are shown in Fig. 5.23. UWB PRF is chosen to be 100 MHz for the signals shown in Fig. 5.23.

Two versions of the dual band sensor node are implemented. The first sensor node has dimensions of 30 mm (L) × 25 mm (W) × 0.7 mm (H); hence, this sensor node is suitable for wearable applications. The second sensor node is circular in design. It is implemented as a combination of two PCBs that can be interconnected with each other in a stack-up configuration. This design has a diameter of 15 mm; hence, it is suitable for both wearable and implantable applications. Both sensor node designs are shown in Fig. 5.24. Figure 5.25 depicts different regions of the PCB design for the first sensor node.

5.2.10 Comparison

Table 5.3 compares specifications of some of the existing WBAN platforms with the suggested sensor node design. Wireless sensor nodes based on narrow band platforms are used widely for WBAN applications. Most of the UWB based designs available in the literature are either limited to Integrated Circuit (IC) based

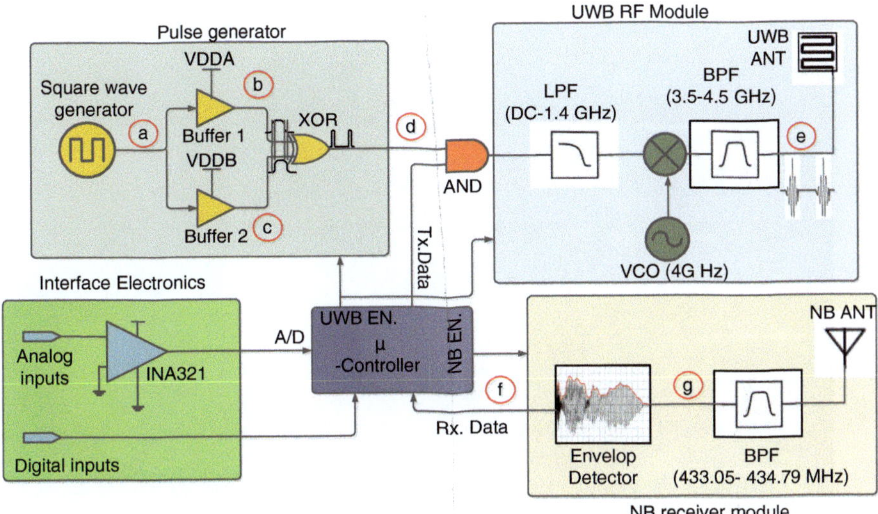

Fig. 5.22 Overall integration of the sensor node

implementations of transmitters/receivers or are not intended for WBAN applications. Hence, comparison in Table 5.3 is limited only to sensor node designs with full implementations, which include wireless transmitters/receivers, microcontrollers and data acquisition electronics.

It can be seen from Table 5.3 that the dual band WBAN sensor node presented in this chapter outperforms other sensor nodes in terms of data rate, power consumption and form factor. This design incorporates the unique advantages provided by UWB, such as possibility of achieving high data rates, low power consumption and simple design while avoiding the complexities introduced by UWB receivers. Because of the use of a narrow band receiver at the sensor node, it is possible to achieve a reliable communication link while consuming low power during data reception.

5.3 Implementation of the Coordinator Node

Coordinator node is responsible for controlling the communication with multiple sensor nodes while maintaining acceptable levels of BER, delay and QoS. It consists of four main component blocks mentioned below:

(1) *IR-UWB receiver front-end*
The IR-UWB receiver front-end down-converts the received UWB pulses creating a base band pulse stream that can be detected using a sampling and data processing unit.

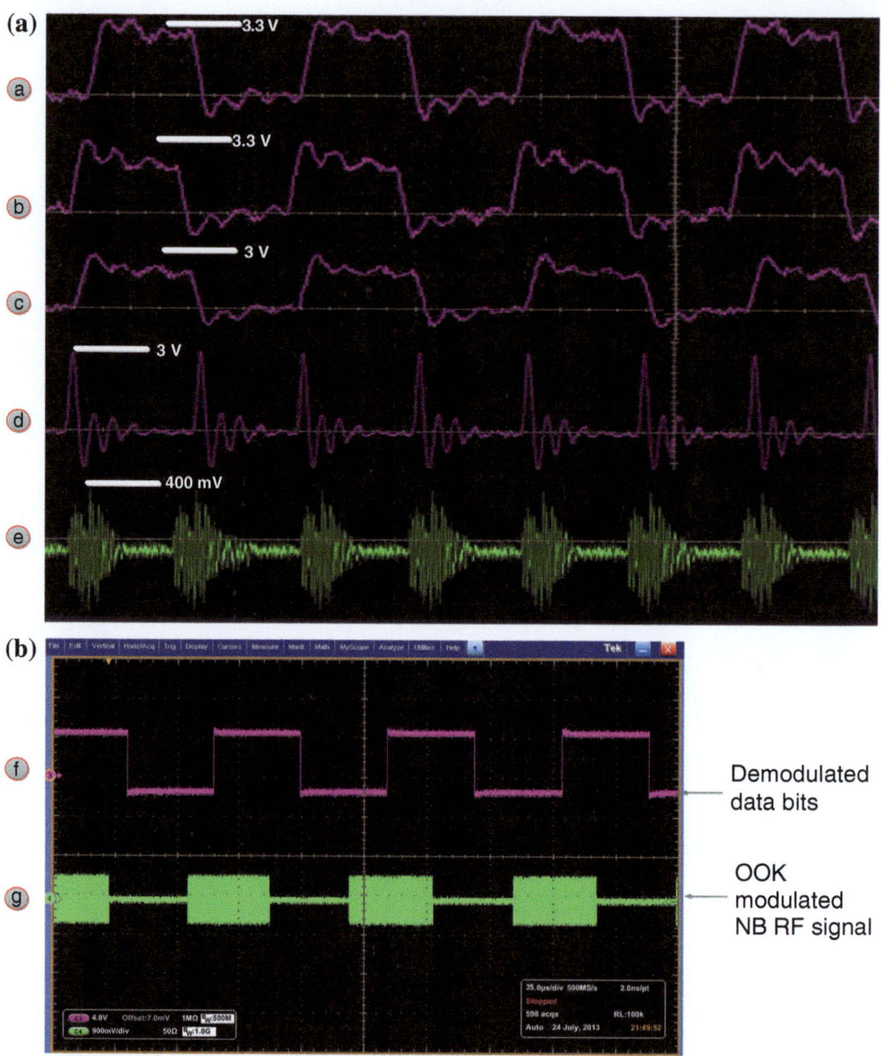

Fig. 5.23 **a** Waveforms taken at various points of the UWB transmitter stion **b** data reception at the narrow band receiver (See Fig. 5.22 for respective reference points related to the waveforms in the sensor node design)

(2) *Narrow band transmitter*

The 433 MHz ISM band transmitter transmits the control messages originated from the FPGA on the narrow band channel.

(3) *Sampling and data processing unit*

The sampling and data processing unit consists of an ADC and a FPGA. It is responsible for the operation of the MAC protocol at the coordinator node.

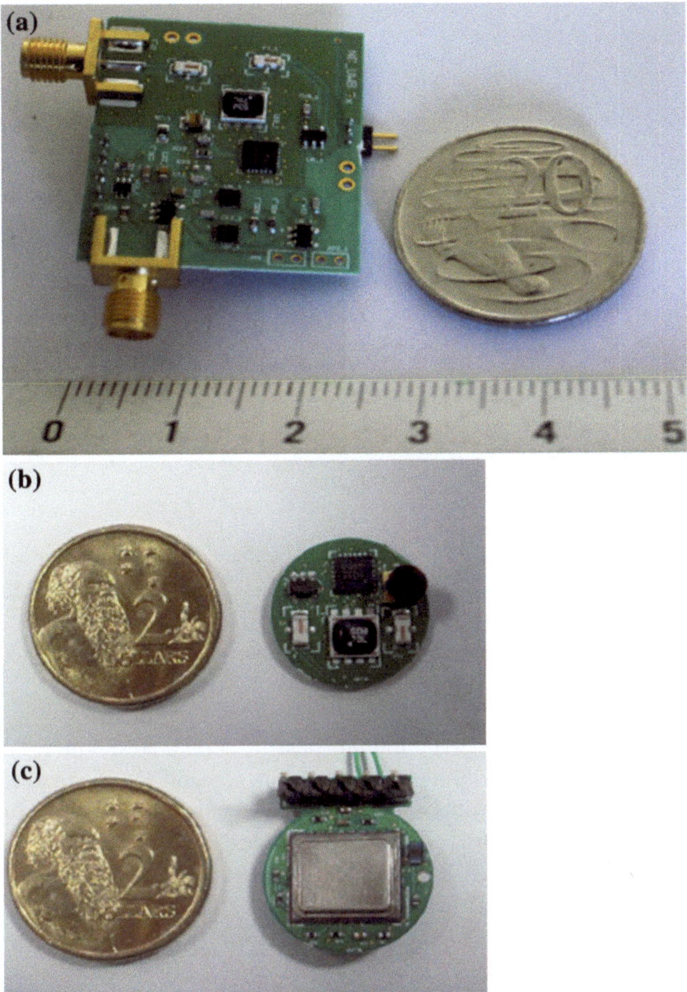

Fig. 5.24 Sensor nodes **a** First sensor design (wearable sensor nodes) **b** Second sensor design - Board 1 **c** Second sensor design- Board 2 (implantable sensor nodes)

(4) *Computer terminal*

The computer terminal communicates with the FPGA and retrieves the data received on the forward (UWB) channel.

The basic block diagram of the coordinator node is shown in Fig. 5.26.

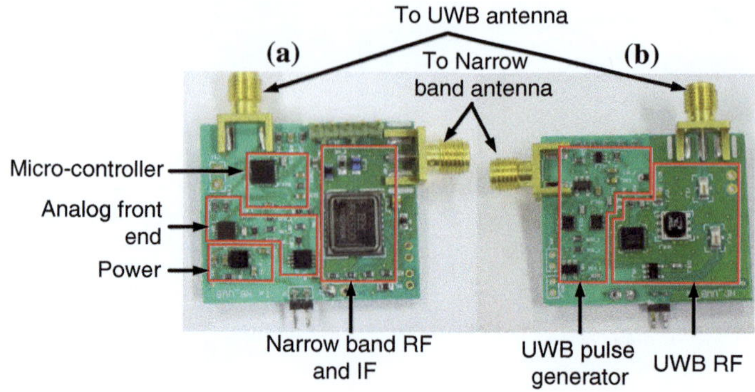

Fig. 5.25 Various sections of the dual band sensor node. **a** Bottom side, **b** Top side

5.3.1 IR-UWB Receiver Front-End

Direct-conversion receiver architecture is utilized for the IR-UWB receiver front-end described herein. Main advantages of using a direct-conversion architecture are the ease of implementation using off-the-shelf components, ability to operate without the use of any timing control and resetting signals as compared to energy detection receivers and small power consumption.

The block diagram of the UWB receiver front-end circuit is shown in Fig. 5.27. UWB signals entering the receiver antenna pass through a BPF with a pass band of 3.5–4.5 GHz in order to eliminate unwanted out-of-band interfering signals. The filtered signal is then amplified by 48 dB using three wideband Low Noise Amplifiers (LNA) before down converting to a baseband signal using a mixer and a VCO operating at 4 GHz. The baseband signal is passed through a LPF with 100 MHz cut-off frequency before going through an analog amplification stage. The LPF acts as a partial integrator and stretches the pulses so that they are easily detectable using the ADC.

Two implementations of the UWB RF front-end are developed based on the receiver architecture shown in Fig. 5.28. The first implementation is realized using plug-in RF components as seen in Fig. 5.28a. The second generation IR-UWB front-end is realized with a PCB using off-the-shelf components (Fig. 5.28b). Table 5.4 depicts major components used in each design.

The LNAs in the first design introduce a gain of 17.27 dB each with a Noise Figure (NF) of 5.44 dB while the LNAs in the second design produce a gain of 16 dB each with a NF of 1.45 dB. Both analog amplifiers produce a gain of 10 dB while the NF for the analog amplifier in first design is 19.2 dB and that of the second design is 16.6 dB. The overall NF for the first design calculated from the Fris formula [26] is 3.55 dB while the second design has an overall NF of 1.41 dB. The mixer in the first design has a conversion loss of 7.22 dB while that of the second design is 7.16 dB. All the band pass filters have an insertion loss of 1 dB while the low pass filters have

Table 5.3 Comparison of WBAN sensor nodes

Model	Company	Frequency	Data rate	Tx. power (dBm)	Physical dimensions (L × W×H) mm / (diameter × H) mm	Power/ current consumption	
						Rx.	Tx.
Mica2 (MPR400)	Crossbow [23]	868/916 MHz	38.4 kbps	−24 to +5	58 × 32 × .7	10 mA at 3.3 V	27 mA at 3.3 V
MicAz	Crossbow [23]	2400–2483 MHz (IEEE 802.15.4)	250 kbps	−24 to 0	58 × 32 × .7	19.7 mA at 3.3 V	17.4 mA at 3.3 V
Mica2DOT	Crossbow [23]	868 /916 MHz and 433 MHz	38.4 kbps	−20 to +10	25 (diameter) × .6	8 mA at 3.3 V	25 mA at 3.3 V
Tmote Sky	Mote iv [24]	2.4 GHz (IEEE 802.15.4)	250 kbps	−25 to 0	66 × 32.6 × .7	21.8 mA at 3 V	19.5 mA at 3 V
MICS node	Monash University [25]	402–405 MHz	76 kbps	−16	30 × 75 × .7	8 mA at 3.3 V	27 mA at 3.3 V
Dual band WBAN node (This design)	Monash University	3.5–4.5 GHz	Up to 5 Mbps	−41.3 dBm/ MHz	30 × 25 × .7 (design 1) and 15 (diameter) × .7 (design 2)	3 mA at 3.3 V	10 mA at 3.3 V

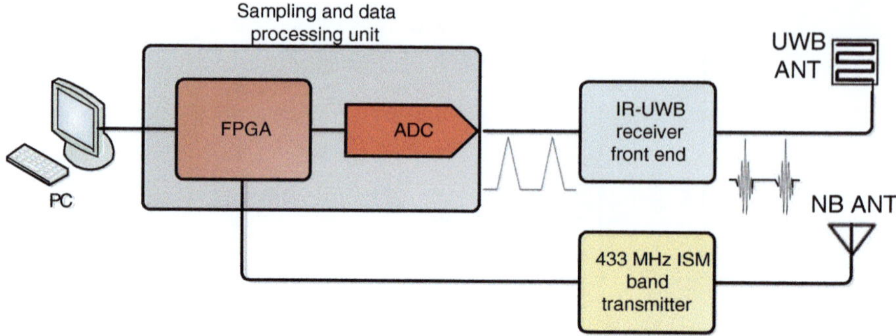

Fig. 5.26 Basic block diagram of the coordinator node

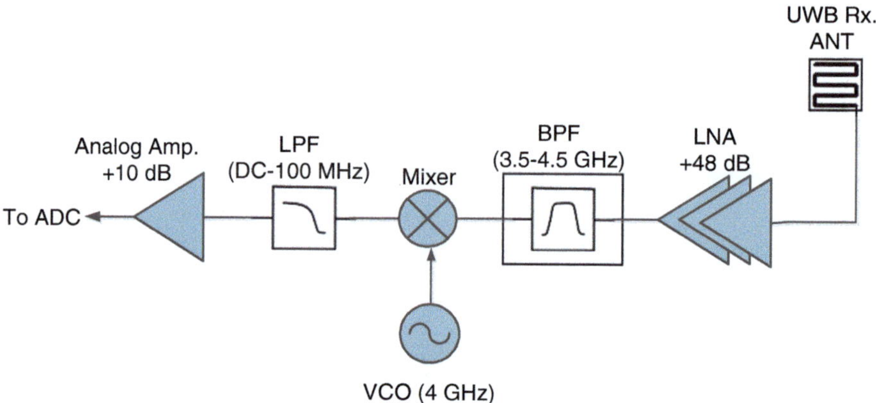

Fig. 5.27 Block diagram of the IR-UWB front-end

an insertion loss of 0.5 dB. The link budgets of both receiver designs for a transmission distance of 1 m and a PRF of 100 MHz are shown in Table 5.5.

The time domain waveforms of the received signals after the mixer stage and after the LPF stage of the receiver (Design 1) for a signal transmitted at a 100 MHz PRF with a transmitter—receiver separation distance of 0.7 m are shown in Fig. 5.29. After the analog amplifier, received UWB pulses are detected using the ADC and the FPGA of the coordinator node. The receive spectrum for each stage of the UWB receiver front-end is shown in Fig. 5.30.

5.3.2 Narrow Band Transmitter

TX5000, which is a 433 MHz ISM transmitter module by RFM [17], is used as the narrow band transmitter of the coordinator node. This off-the-shelf transmitter module can transmit data using both OOK and ASK modulation schemes. Narrow

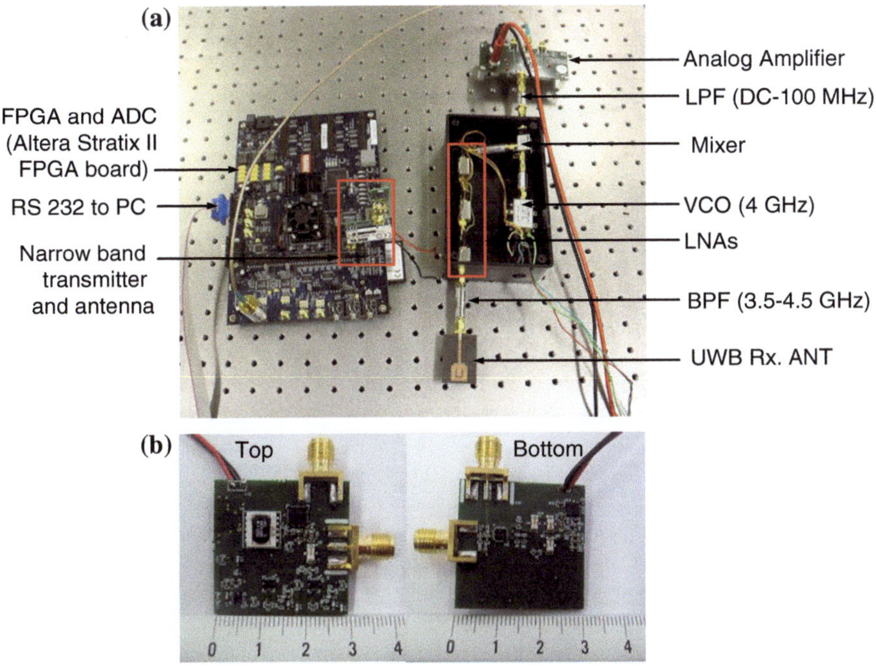

Fig. 5.28 **a** Components of the coordinator node with UWB receiver front-end made out of plug-in RF components **b** UWB receiver front-end implemented on a PCB

Table 5.4 Components for UWB RF front-end designs

Functional block	Design 1	Design 2
Mixer	ZX05-63LH-S+ [15]	MACA-63H+ [15]
BPF	VBFZ-4000-S+ [15]	BFCN-4440+ [15]
LPF	VLF-105+ [13]	LFCN-1400+ [15]
VCO	ZX95-4100-S+ [15]	HMC391LP4 [16]
LNA	MGA-665P8 [27]	ZX60-5916 M-S+ [15]
Analog amplifier	THS4508 [19]	AD8000 [11]

band transmitter module directly receives data from FPGA and transmits using the 433 MHz ISM band. This is mainly used to transmit beacon messages and control messages to the sensor nodes. The data rate of the transmitter can be varied from 19.2 kbps down to 4 kbps; hence, it is suitable for the transmission of low data rate beacon and control messages.

Table 5.5 Link budget analysis for the two UWB receiver designs

Parameter	Value	
	Design 1	Design 2
Frequency	3.5–4.5 GHz	
Throughput (R_b)	5 Mbps	
Signal bandwidth (B)	1 GHz	
Transmitter implementation loss (L_{Tx})	5 dB	
Average Tx. Power ($P_{Tx} = -41.3$ dBm/MHz $+ 10\log(B/1$ MHz$) - L_{Tx}$)	-16.3 dBm	
Tx antenna gain (G_T)	0 dBi	
Average path loss (PL) at 1 m [28]	55 dB	
Rx antenna gain (G_R)	0 dBi	
Average Rx power ($P_{Rx} = P_{Tx} - PL$)	-71.3 dBm	
Thermal noise ($N_0 = -174$ dBm/Hz $+ 10\log$ (B)	-84 dBm	
Noise figure (NF)	3.55 dB	1.41 dB
Minimum signal to noise ratio requirement (SNR_{min})	12 dB	
Receiver implementation loss (L_{Rx})	9 dB	
Processing gain ($G_p = 10\log (B/R_b)$)	23 dB	
Receiver sensitivity at 1 m ($P_{R,min} = N_0 + NF + SNR_{min} + L_{Rx} - G_p$)	-82.45 dBm	-84.59 dBm
Link margin ($M = P_R - P_{R,min}$)	11.15 dB	13.29 dB

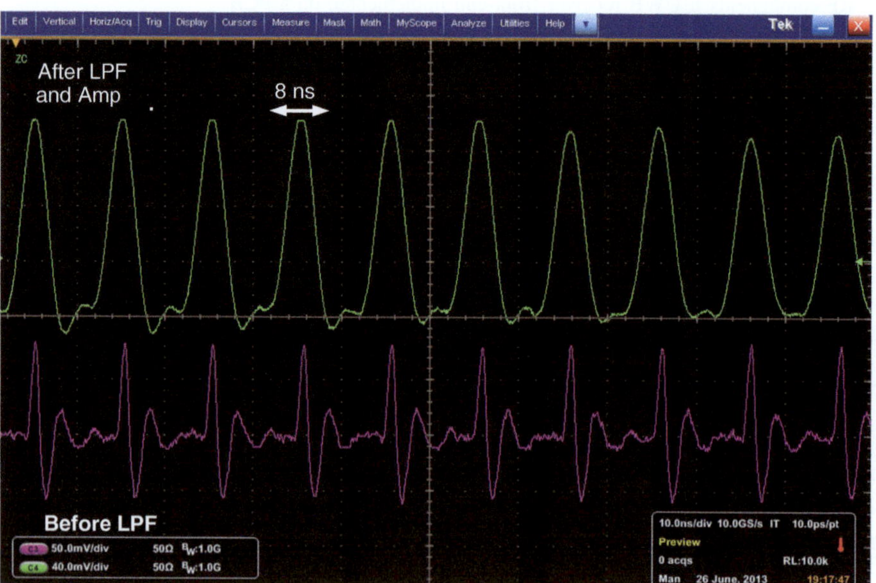

Fig. 5.29 Received UWB signals

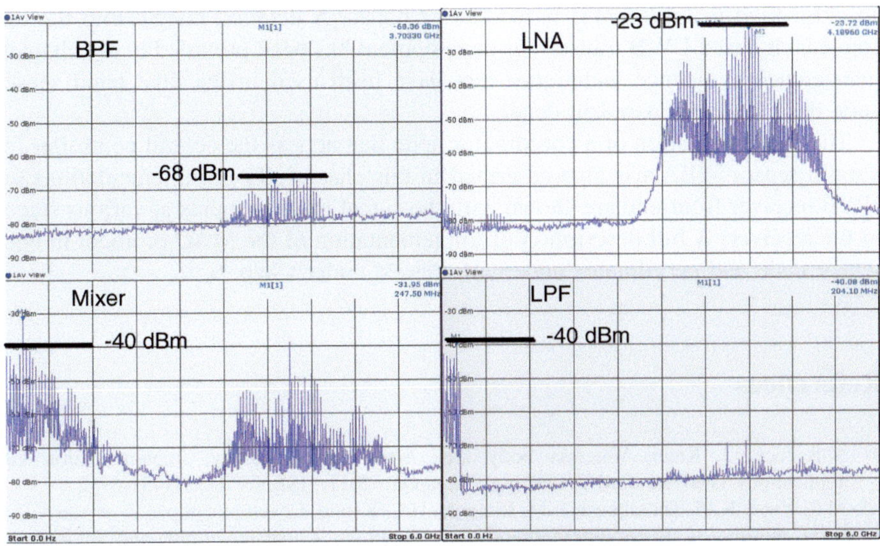

Fig. 5.30 Spectrums for various receive stages of the UWB front-end

5.3.3 Sampling and Data Processing Unit

Altera Stratix II FPGA board [29] is used for data sampling and MAC protocol operation at the coordinator node. The FPGA board has an on-board ADC module that can be operated at a sampling rate of 100 MHz and with a resolution of 12 bits/sample. Broadened UWB pulses that come out from the analog amplifier of the UWB frond-end are sampled using this ADC module and compared against a threshold level using a comparator that is programmed into the FPGA module in order to determine the presence of a pulse. A detailed description of the pulse detection method and the MAC protocol implementation in the FPGA module is given in Chap. 6. FPGA module communicates with a computer terminal that is used to store and display data.

5.4 Conclusion

The hardware implementation of a dual band communication system for WBAN applications is discussed in this chapter. Even though many IC based implementations of the UWB pulse generators and receivers can be found in the literature, only few discuss the full implementation of a WBAN system. Even fewer studies in the literature have paid attention to resolving the complexities caused by using a UWB receiver at the power stringent sensor nodes. This chapter discusses the full design of a dual band sensor node implemented using off-the-shelf components as an alternative to fully UWB based sensor nodes. A detailed insight into the up-conversion based UWB transmitter development has been provided in the chapter. Interference avoidance techniques that have been used in the dual band sensor node design are discussed in detail.

The implementation of a coordinator node that acts as the central controller for a multi sensor WBAN is also described in this chapter. Two implementations for UWB receiver front-end are shown with the signal measurements at various stages of the receiver. A full description of implementation of the MAC protocol in both sensor node and coordinator node is discussed under Chap. 6.

References

1. M.R.Yuce, J. Khan, Wireless body area networks: technology, implementation and applications. (Pan Stanford Publishing, Singapore, 2011), ISBN 978-981-431-6712
2. M.R. Yuce, K.M. Thotahewa, J.-M. Redoute, H.C. Keong, Development of low-power UWB body sensors, in *IEEE International Symposium on Communications and Information Technologies (ISCIT)*, pp. 143–148, Oct 2012
3. M.R. Yuce, H.C. Keong, M. Chae, Wideband communication for implantable and wearable systems. IEEE Trans. Microw. Theory Tech. **57,** Part 2, 2597–2604 (2009)
4. K.M.S. Thotahewa, J.-M.Redoute, M.R. Yuce, Implementation of ultra-wideband (UWB) sensor nodes for WBAN applications, Ultra-Wideband and 60 GHz communications for biomedical applications. (Springer, New York, 2014)
5. K.M. Thotahewa, J.-M. Redoute, M.R. Yuce, Implementation of a dual band body sensor node, in *IEEE MTT-S International Microwave Workshop Series on RF and Wireless Technologies for Biomedical and Healthcare (IMWS-Bio2013)*, 2013
6. K.M. Thotahewa, J.-M. Redoute, M.R. Yuce, A low-power, wearable, dual-band wireless body area network system: development and experimental evaluation, submitted
7. N.R. Mahapatra, A. Tareen, S.V. Garimella, Comparison and analysis of delay elements. IEEE Midwest Circuits Syst. Symp. **2,** 473–476 (2002)
8. M. Cavallaro, T. Copani, G. Palmisano, A Gaussian pulse generator for millimeter-wave applications. IEEE Trans. Circuits Syst. I Regul. Pap. **57,** 1212–1220 (2010)
9. Y.P. Nakache, A.F. Molisch, Spectral shape of UWB signals—influence of modulation format, multiple access scheme and pulse shape, IEEE Veh. Technol. Conf. **4,** 2510–2514 (2003)
10. http://www.linear.com/ 2014
11. http://www.analog.com 2014
12. http://www.fairchildsemi.com/ 2014
13. E. Bogatin, *Signal Integrity—Simplified*, 1st edn. (Prentice Hall, New Jersey, 2004)
14. J. Colli-Vignarelli, C. Dehollain, A discrete-components impulse-radio ultrawide-band (IR-UWB) transmitter. IEEE Trans. Microw. Theory Tech. **59,** 1141–1146 (2011)
15. http://www.minicircuits.com 2014
16. http://www.hittite.com 2014
17. http://www.rfm.com 2014
18. http://www.microchip.com 2014
19. http://www.ti.com 2014
20. J. Davis, *High-Speed Digital System Design*, 1st edn. (Morgan and Claypool, California, 2006)

21. C. Chastang, C. Gautier, M. Brizoux, A. Grivon, V. Tissier, A. Amedeo, F. Costa, Electrical behavior of stacked microvias integration technologies for multi-gigabits applications using 3D simulation, in *15th IEEE Workshop on Signal Propagation on Interconnects*, pp. 65–68, 2011
22. B.C. Wadell (1991) *Transmission line design handbook.* (Artech House, London, 1991), pp. 79–80
23. http://www.xbow.com/ 2014
24. http://www.eecs.harvard.edu/ ~ konrad/projects/shimmer/references/tmote-sky-datasheet.pdf 2014
25. M.R. Yuce, Implementation of wireless body area networks for healthcare systems. Sens. Actuators A Phys. **162**, 116–129 (2010)
26. B. Razavi, *RF Microelectronics* (Prentice-Hall, Upper Saddle River, 2006)
27. http://www.avagotech.com 2014
28. IEEE P802.15-02/490r1-SG3a, Channel Modeling Sub-committee Report Final, Feb 2003
29. http://www.altera.com/ 2014

Chapter 6
System Implementation and Evaluation of an Energy Efficient UWB-Based MAC Protocol for Wireless Body Area Networks

Abstract A Wireless Body Area Network (WBAN) should operate with minimum power consumption while providing reliable data transmission. This chapter describes system implementation of a Medium Access control (MAC) protocol for WBAN applications. A WBAN is implemented using four UWB WBAN sensor nodes and a coordinator node in order to evaluate the real-time performance of the MAC protocol. A detailed description of the firmware implementation of the MAC protocol is given including code examples of a Field Programmable Gate Array (FPGA) based firmware implementation. Performance parameters of the network are evaluated for various communication scenarios. This chapter also presents the power consumption measurements of UWB WBAN sensor nodes during real-time network operation. These power measurements represent the detailed power efficiency of both hardware design and MAC protocol design.

Keywords UWB · Power consumption · WBAN packet frame · Dual-band · MAC · Firmware implementation · FPGA · Pulse synchronization · Bit detection · BER · Energy consumption

6.1 Introduction

Design and implementation of an efficient MAC protocol plays a vital role in reducing power consumption and increasing reliability of data transmission. It is vital to utilize the unique physical properties of an UWB signal, such as the possibility to send multiple numbers of pulses to represent a data bit, in order to improve the system performance [1–3]. The performance of an UWB communication link is greatly affected by the effects of body motion [4, 5]. The ability of a MAC protocol to adjust to such dynamic channel conditions plays a vital role in providing a reliable communication link.

The dual-band MAC protocol described in Chap. 3 utilizes the physical layer properties of UWB signal to form a cross layer MAC design. It accommodates

K. M. S. Thotahewa et al., *Ultra Wideband Wireless Body Area Networks*,   117
DOI: 10.1007/978-3-319-05287-8_6,

reliable and power efficient multi sensor communication between dual-band sensor nodes and coordinator node [6, 7]. This chapter describes the implementation and evaluation of this dual-band MAC protocol in a hardware based system [7, 8]. The MAC protocol is adjusted to suit the implementation using available hardware platforms. Differences between the simulations described in Chap. 3 and system implementation of the MAC protocol that is discussed in this chapter are listed below;

1. On-Off-Keying (OOK) modulation is used instead of Binary Pulse Position Modulation (BPPM) considering the ease of hardware implementation of OOK modulation, and its similar performance to BPPM.
2. A direct conversion receiver that down-converts the received IR-UWB pulses using a mixer and apply low pass filtering to broaden the down-converted pulses is used instead of an energy detection based receiver architecture used for simulations in Chap. 3. This is mainly due to the ease of implementation of the direct conversion receiver using off-the-shelf components, ability to operate without the use of any control signals as compared to energy detection receiver, and small power consumption.
3. Data packet lengths and time slot durations of the super frame are adjusted according to the communication scenarios presented in this chapter.

Apart from these differences, implementation of the MAC protocol is similar to the MAC protocol discussed in Chap. 3. A full system implementation, including a FPGA based firmware implementation is presented in this chapter. Important algorithms used in the MAC protocol are described in terms of flow diagrams and Very High Speed Integrated Circuit Hardware Description Language (VHDL) code implementation examples. This chapter also presents the experimental evaluation of the dual-band MAC protocol in terms of Bit Error Rate (BER), initialization delay and power consumption.

6.2 Development of Packet Structure

Data communication between dual-band sensor nodes and the coordinator node occurs using the beacon enabled super frame structure described in Chap. 3. Data and control packets are sent within an allocated super frame time slot in order to realize a reliable communication link. A maximum super frame time slot duration of 100 µs is used for data transmission of continuous sensor nodes and that of periodic sensor nodes is chosen as 50 µs. These timing parameters ensure that sensor nodes transmit at a duty cycle that is less than 18.75 % based on a super frame duration of 1 ms, enabling sensor nodes to utilize the maximum full bandwidth peak power (refer Chap. 3). Data packet structures used in the system implementation of the MAC protocol is shown in Fig. 6.1.

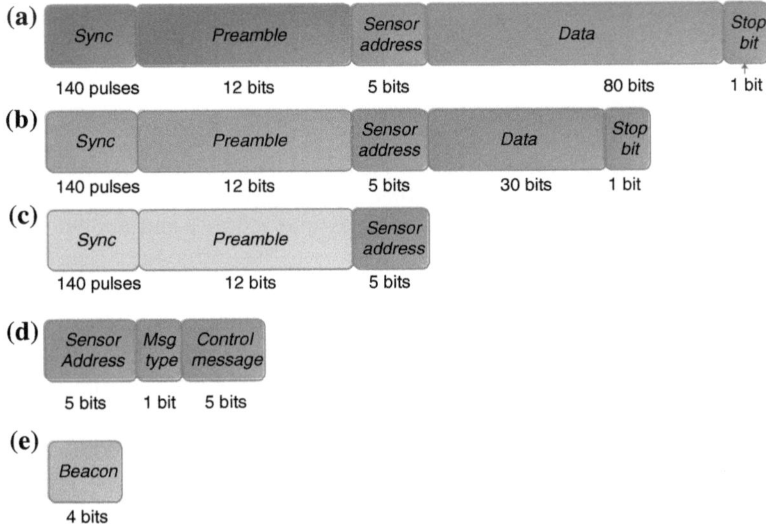

Fig. 6.1 **a** Transmit data packet for continuous sensors on the IR-UWB link, **b** transmit data packet for periodic sensors on the IR-UWB link, **c** initialization request packet, **d** receive control packet on the narrowband link, **e** beacon

Transmit data packet structure is modified from the one used in Chap. 3 considering the data generation capabilities of the dual-band sensor nodes. The micro-controller used in the dual-band sensor nodes is capable of generating data bits that can be modulated with a minimum of 20 Pulses Per Bit (PPB) when the IR-UWB pulse generator module is operating at a Pulse Repetitive Frequency (PRF) of 100 MHz. This results in a maximum achievable instantaneous data rate of 5 Mbps. Hence, 20 PPB is chosen as the minimum allowable PPB for the UWB transmission. Maximum allowable PPB value is chosen to be 100 PPB considering the lower bounds of data rate requirements. 140 IR-UWB pulses are sent during the *Sync* portion of transmit packet by all the sensor nodes irrespective of the number of PPB allocated for the data transmission. This is used for synchronization of the Analog to Digital Converter (ADC) sampling as discussed in a following section. Initialization packets are used during the first two time slots of the super frame structure for the purpose of contention based sensor initialization. Control packets on the narrowband channel are mainly used for sensor initialization and dynamically assigning PPB value for each sensor node during changing channel conditions. Beacon packets are used for the super frame synchronization. They are sent on the narrowband channel that operates at a data rate of 19.2 kbps. All the bit lengths used in packet structures are calculated based on factors, such as the amount of data that should be transmitted using a particular packet, maximum allowable PPB value that is to be used in each packet transmitted on the UWB channel, and maximum allowable duty cycle for data transmission using each packet.

6.3 Cross Layer MAC Protocol Implementation at Sensor Node

A sensor node synchronises to the super frame structure used in the MAC protocol by listening to the beacon packets transmitted on the narrowband channel. A super frame structure consists of two initialization time slots at the beginning of the super frame. Position of these initialization time slots is pre-known to all the sensor nodes. This is determined using a time delay measured with reference to the end of beacon reception period. At sensor initialization, a sensor node transmits an initialization request message using the packet structure shown in Fig. 6.1c and starts a time-out operation in order to determine whether the sensor node gets an initialization respond from the coordinator node within a given amount of time. A unique pre-programmed sensor address is used in the initialization request packet. Sensor node then waits until the reception of initialization acknowledgement packet that contains transmit time slot and PPB value assigned for that sensor node. If a time-out occurs without receiving the initialization acknowledgement packet, sensor node then retransmits an initialization request message during the initialization slots of the following super frame. The maximum number of initialization attempts is limited to 10. After initialization, sensor node transmits data in the pre-allocated time slot and listens to any BER correction control messages on the narrowband receiver. Implementation of the BER correction procedure in discussed in the following sub section. Figure 6.2 depicts the overall operation of sensor node control program that is implemented in the micro-controller module.

6.4 Cross Layer MAC Protocol Implementation at the Coordinator Node

The coordinator node is responsible for organizing and controlling the data communication of sensor nodes. Main operations carried out by the control program of coordinator node are listed below;

1. IR-UWB pulse synchronization
2. Data bit detection and packet synchronization
3. Dynamic BER detection and feedback control.

6.4.1 Pulse Synchronization for IR-UWB WBAN Communication

IR-UWB pulse detection is done by an ADC module and a Field Programmable Gate Array (FPGA) that are integral parts of the coordinator node. The ADC module samples the broadened base band pulse stream that is generated by IR-UWB front-end. Pulse detection program is implemented in the FPGA module.

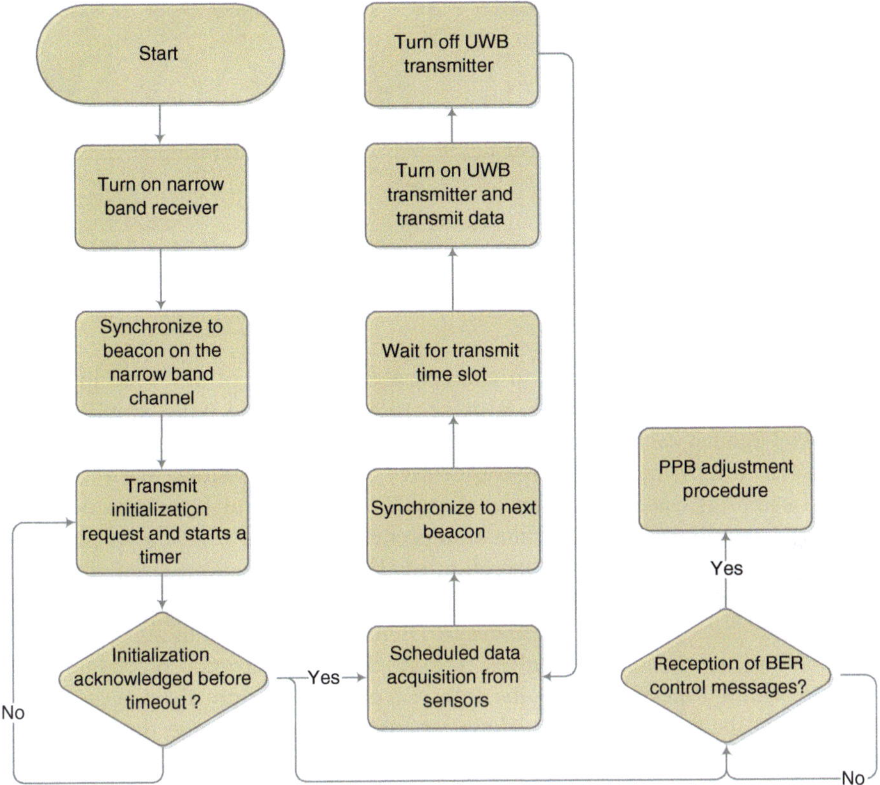

Fig. 6.2 Operation of the sensor node control program

Stratix II FPGA development board [9] is used as the sampling and data processing module of coordinator node. Stratix II FPGA development board has an
on-board ADC module that can sample the base band pulses at a sampling speed of
100 MHz and with a resolution of 12 bits per sample. Pulse detection and synchronization algorithm is programmed into the FPGA module. Pulse detection
program in the FPGA operates a Digital Phase Locked Loop (DPLL) that generates six clocks with programmable delays with respect to a reference clock.
Function of the pulse synchronization algorithm implemented in the FPGA module
is to determine the ADC sampling clock that samples at the peak of received UWB
pulses. For example, consider a UWB system that operates at a 100 MHz PRF. In
this case, the UWB front-end will generate a base band pulse stream with pulses
that are 8 ns wide and 10 ns apart from each other. Six clocks having a delay of
1.67 ns (phase difference of 60°) from each other and a clock frequency of
100 MHz are generated by the DPLL of the FPGA program. These clocks sample
the UWB pulse stream sequentially. Each clock samples 10 consecutive UWB
pulses and stores the recorded pulse amplitudes as a summation. Ten sample

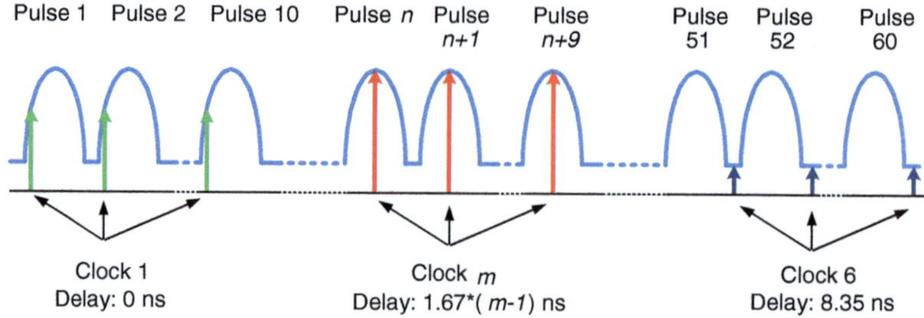

Fig. 6.3 Pulse detection using different sampling clocks

pulses for each clock are used to compensate for effects of any time jitters that might occur in the received UWB pulse stream. Recorded pulse amplitudes are compared against each other after all the clocks have finished sampling the pulse stream (i.e. after a period of 60 consecutive pulses). The clock that records the highest sampling value is chosen as the ADC sampling clock for data detection. The ADC sampling clock determination procedure occurs within *Sync* portion of the transmit packet structure. Operation of the above-mentioned sampling technique is shown in Figs. 6.3 and 6.4.

IR-UWB pulse synchronization ensures that an optimum sampling clock is used to sample the received UWB pulses. The clock synchronization procedure has to operate within *Sync* portion of the transmit packet structure for accurate determination of the sampling clock. However, start of a super frame time slot might not always be aligned with time of arrival of the packet structure. Hence, a procedure has to be developed in order to avoid the clock inaccuracies due to the delay between start of the super frame time slot and packet arrival time. This is achieved in the following manner.

The FPGA program defines an initial amplitude threshold value for detecting the presence of a pulse. A pulse is considered present if the recorded pulse amplitude by the ADC module exceeds the threshold value. The FPGA module can detect amplitudes ranging from -1 to $+1$ V with a resolution of 5 mV. Considering the fact that received pulses after the UWB front-end possess a positive amplitude, 10 mV is chosen as the initial threshold level in the pulse detection algorithm. Choosing the lowest possible threshold level for data detection eliminates the requirement for changing the threshold level according to the distance between a sensor node and the coordinator node. *Sync* portion of the transmit packet is followed by a 12 bit preamble sequence that is chosen to be "010010110100".

As described earlier, the ADC module samples 10 baseband pulses using each clock (initial detections) in a sequential manner at the start of a super frame time slot that has been allocated for the data transmission of a particular sensor node (Fig. 6.5a). This is carried out without prior knowledge of the position of *Sync* portion within the received packet structure. The recorded pulse amplitudes for each clock are compared against the initial threshold value in order to determine

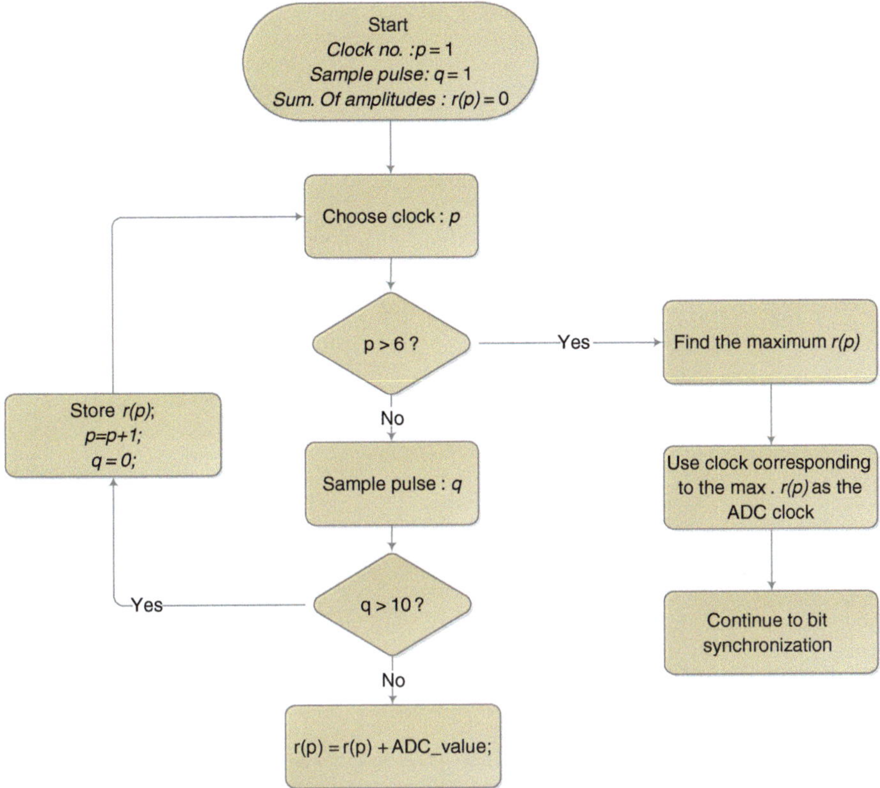

Fig. 6.4 Algorithm for determining the sampling clock

the presence of a pulse (For the ease of notation, presence of a pulse is denoted as P_1 and absence of a pulse is denoted as P_0 herein). The FPGA program waits until the first instance where one of the sampling clocks records five P_1 s out of the ten pulses sampled by the ADC. The occurrence of the latter event records arrival of the packet. Receiver sampling clock is in sub optimal synchronization at this moment. A full clock synchronization procedure is carried out according to the algorithm shown in Fig. 6.4 after the detection of initial pulses in order to achieve the optimal sampling clock. Figure 6.5 depicts the VHDL code implementation of the pulse synchronization process.

Sync portion of the transmit packet consists of 140 pulse periods whereas the clock synchronization period described in Fig. 6.4 only requires 60 pulse periods. The extra number of pulses within the *Sync* portion of the packet structure is utilized to assure that a full set of 60 pulses can be used for clock synchronization (Fig. 6.6b, c). Clock synchronization is followed by the preamble detection. This is described in the following subsection.

```vhdl
library ieee;
use ieee.std_logic_1164.all;
use ieee.std_logic_arith.all;

entity PULSE_SYNC is

    port(
        clk : in std_logic; -- FPGA clock
        ADC_in : in std_logic_vector(11 downto 0); --12 bit input from ADC
        CLK_sel : out std_logic_vector(2 downto 0);-- Sampling clock to ADC module
        );
end entity PULSE_SYNC;

architecture SYNCArch of PULSE_SYNC is
    type Sync_block_type is (block1, block2, block3,
    block4, block5, block6);  -- Six Sync blocks for six sampling clocks
    signal Sync_block : Sync_block_type := block1;
    signal rxdata : std_logic_vector(11 downto 0);
    signal pulse_cnt : std_logic_vector (3 downto 0) := "0000"; --Count upto ten consecutive pulses

    SYNC : process(clk)

        variable ADC_store1,ADC_store2,ADC_store3,ADC_store4
        ,ADC_store5,ADC_store6,ADCmax : std_logic_vector(20 downto 0) ;
        variable opt_clk : std_logic_vector (2 downto 0); -- Optimum clock to be used in pulse detection
        variable ADC_max : std_logic_vector(20 downto 0):= "000000000000000000000";

        begin

            if clk'event and clk = '1' then

                case Sync_block is

                    when block1 =>
                        CLK_sel <= "000"; -- Use clock no.1 for sampling 10 consecutive pulses (See Fig. 6-3)
                        rxdata <= ADC_in;
                        ADC_store1 := ADC_store1 + rxdata;
                        pulse_cnt <= Pulse_cnt + 1;

                        if pulse_cnt < "1001" then -- If number of pulses sampled are less than 10
                            Sync_block <= block1;
                        else                    -- When number of pulses sampled equal to 10
                            opt_clk := "000";  --Assign Clock no. 1 as the optimum sampling clock
                            ADC_max := ADC_store1; -- Assign ADCStore1 as the maximum recorded cumuative_
                                            -- _ADC sampling value
                            ADC_store1 := "000000000000000000000";
                            pulse_cnt <= "0000";
                            Sync_block <= block2;
                        end if;
                    when block2 =>
                        CLK_sel <= "001"; -- Use clock no.2 for sampling 10 consecutive pulses (See Fig. 6-3)
                        rxdata <= ADC_in;
                        ADC_store2 := ADC_store2 + rxdata;
                        pulse_cnt <= Pulse_cnt + 1;

                        if pulse_cnt < "1001" then -- If number of pulses sampled are less than 10
                            Sync_block <= block2;
                        else if ADC_max < ADC_store2 then   -- If Clock no.2 records a larger cumulative_
                                            -- _sampling value than the previous maximum
                            opt_clk := "001";   --Assign Clock no. 2 as the optimum sampling clock
                            ADC_max := ADC_store2;
                            ADC_store2 := "000000000000000000000";
                            pulse_cnt <= "0000";
                            Sync_block <= block3;
                        else                -- Else keep the previous maximum ADC and sampling clock
                                            --and move to next block
                            ADC_store2 := "000000000000000000000";
                            pulse_cnt <= "0000";
                            Sync_block <= block3;
                        end if;

                        --contd--
                        --contd--
                    when block6 =>
                        CLK_sel <= "101"; -- Use clock no.6 for sampling 10 consecutive pulses (See Fig. 6-3)

                        rxdata <= ADC_in;
                        ADC_store6 := ADC_store6 + rxdata;
                        pulse_cnt <= Pulse_cnt + 1;

                        if pulse_cnt < "1001" then
                            Sync_block <= block6;
                        else if ADC_max < ADC_store6 then
                            ADC_max := "000000000000000000000";
                            ADC_store6 := "000000000000000000000";
                            pulse_cnt <= "0000";
                        else
                            CLK_sel <= opt_clk; -- Assign the optimum clock found as the ADC sampling_
                                            -- _clock for rest of the packet (In case it is Clock. no 6_
                                            -- _keep the CLK_sel assigned at the begining of this block)
                            ADC_max := "000000000000000000000";
                            ADC_store6 := "000000000000000000000";
                            pulse_cnt <= "0000";
                        end if;

                end case;
        end process SYNC;
end SYNCArch;
```

Fig. 6.5 VHDL code example for pulse synchronization of the receiver algorithm

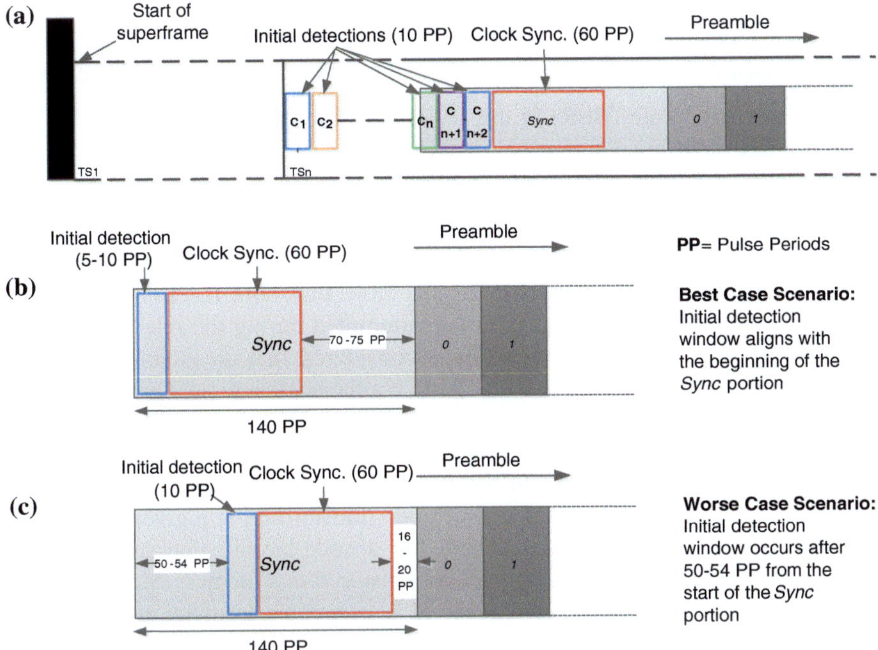

Fig. 6.6 Alignment of clock synchronization period and *Sync* portion

6.4.2 Packet Synchronization and Bit Detection

After the clock synchronization period, the FPGA program waits until the arrival of the first '*0*' of preamble sequence. Optimum clock determined during the clock synchronization period is used together with the initial threshold value in order to determine the presence of a pulse. After clock synchronization, the FPGA program waits until 10 consecutive P_0 s are detected irrespective of the PPB value used for data transmission (PPB values can vary from 20 to 100 PPB for UWB communication described in this chapter). These 10 consecutive P_0 s correspond to the beginning of the first '*0*' bit within the 12-bit preamble sequence. Use of 10 consecutive P_0 s avoids the errors that can be generated due to miss detection of pulses. At the reception of ten consecutive P_0 s, the FPGA program locks into the preamble code by setting the start of bit detection period to the time of detection for first recorded P_0. After locking into the start of the preamble sequence, the FPGA program moves on to detection of the preamble bits using the assigned PPB value for a particular sensor node. A bit is considered to be '1' if number of pulse detections (P_1 s) during a bit period is more than half the number of assigned PPB value (for sensor initialization packets sensor nodes use a pre-known 100 PPB while the data communication that occur after sensor initialization use a PPB value assigned by the coordinator node); otherwise it's assumed to be zero.

Correct detection of preamble assures that the initial threshold value is sufficient for bit detection and that the clock synchronization occurs at the start of packet structure. Incorrect detection of preamble can occur due to two reasons;

1. High Bit Error Rate (BER) in the UWB channel.
2. Initial threshold level sitting below the noise level of received signal.

The program at the receiver is designed to differentiate between these two scenarios in the following manner. If the initial threshold level is below the noise level of the received signal, the preamble detection procedure records all P_1 pulses during a preamble detection period. In this case, threshold level is increased by 1 mV step and clock synchronization is reattempted during the relevant time slot of the next super frame. Otherwise, it is considered that an incorrect preamble detection occurs due to a high BER. BER compensation procedure is discussed under the following sub section.

A successful preamble detection is followed by the bit detection. The coordinator node has prior knowledge of the parameters, such as the PPB value and the threshold level, assigned for each sensor node transmitting at a given time slot of the super frame. These properties are used to decode the bits that are transmitted by the sensor nodes. Decoded data packets are stored in a memory card attached to the FPGA board, and sent on request to a computer terminal using a serial communication.

6.4.3 BER Performance Control Using and the Feedback in the Network for Reliable Data Communication

The coordinator node detects the BER for all the sensor nodes that transmit data in real time using the preamble code and a known 10 bit data pattern of '*1011001110*' spread among data bits within a transmit packet. Coordinator node attempts to keep the BER threshold at 10^{-4} or the closest possible value using the BER compensation procedure described in Chap. 3. When an erroneous bit is detected for a particular sensor node in either the preamble code or known bit pattern embedded in data section of the packet, data detection program starts counting the number of bits received for that particular sensor node from there onwards. If a second erroneous bit is detected before 10,000 bit counts, the bit counter is reset and feedback message is sent via the narrowband feedback path requesting for an increase in the PPB value for that particular sensor node. In case where an erroneous bit is not found, bit counter is reset after reaching the 10000 bit counts. This BER compensation procedure is further discussed under Chap. 3. Overall operation of the data detection procedure for a particular sensor node is shown in Fig. 6.7.

Rest of the MAC protocol operates in the same way as described in Chap. 3. It uses the beacon enabled super frame structure shown in Chap. 3. Super frame

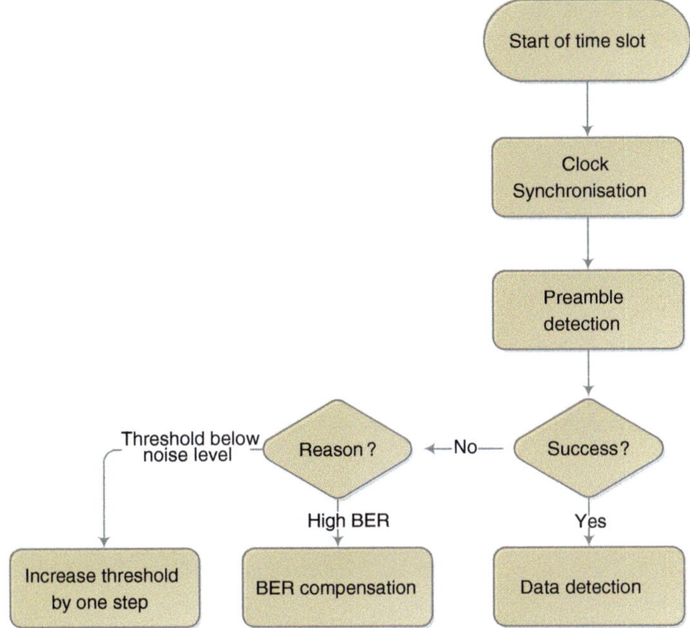

Fig. 6.7 Overall operation of data detection

duration of 1 ms is used for all the sensor communications. Continuous sensors transmit in Guaranteed Time Slots (GTS) with a duration of 100 µs, while periodic sensors transmit during Contention Access Period (CAP) within a time slot duration of 50 µs. Figure 6.8 depicts a decoded bit stream by the FPGA module using the data detection methodology described above.

6.5 A WBAN Implementation: Multi Sensor ECG and Temperature Monitoring System

A multi sensor ECG and temperature monitoring system is set up in order to demonstrate the overall operation of the MAC protocol [8]. Three sensor nodes are used for ECG monitoring while one sensor node is used for the periodic temperature monitoring. Sensor nodes that transmit ECG data use GTS for continuous data transmission while the sensor node that transmits temperature data uses CAP for periodic data transmission. The period of data transmission for the temperature sensor is chosen to be 10 s. All the sensor nodes are placed on-body of a single user while the coordinator node is placed outside the body. Distance between body and receiver antenna is kept at 70 cm for the demonstrated experimental set up.

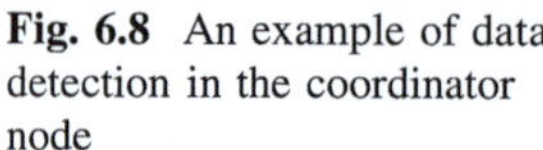

Fig. 6.8 An example of data detection in the coordinator node

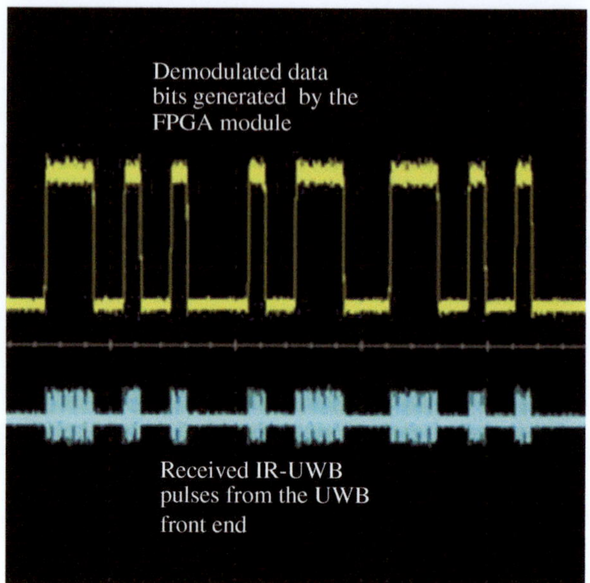

Sensor nodes are arranged such that their antennas are facing towards antennas of the coordinator node.

Two ECG electrodes are used per continuous sensor node in order to obtain ECG measurements. ECG signals are amplified and filtered using the analog front-end circuitry in the sensor node. Inbuilt ADC of the micro-controller is used for sampling the amplified ECG signal. Sampling of the ECG signals is carried out during the sleep mode operation in between the data transmission. ECG signals are sampled at a sampling rate of 8 kHz with a resolution of 10 bits per sample. This generates 70 bits of ECG data per sampling cycle. Sampled data is buffered at the micro-controller and sent during the next data transmission time slot using the continuous data packet structure shown in Fig. 6.1a. An on-board temperature sensor that generates a 10-bit digital data output is used for the purpose of temperature monitoring. Two temperature data samples buffered and transmitted every 10 s using the periodic data packet structure shown in Fig. 6.1b.

Received data is stored at the coordinator node, and transmitted to a computer terminal on request using serial communication. Data gathering and displaying is handled using a program developed in Matlab [10]. A software based notch filter is used to filter out the 50 Hz noise in the received ECG signal. Figure 6.9 depicts the experimental set up used for the monitoring system. Figure 6.10 shows the monitoring interface developed using Matlab. The random initialization of the sensor nodes can be clearly observed in ECG waveforms shown in Fig. 6.10.

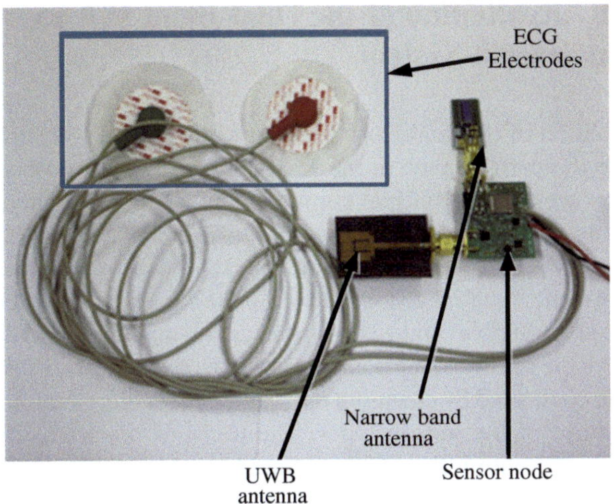

Fig. 6.9 Sensor node used for ECG monitoring

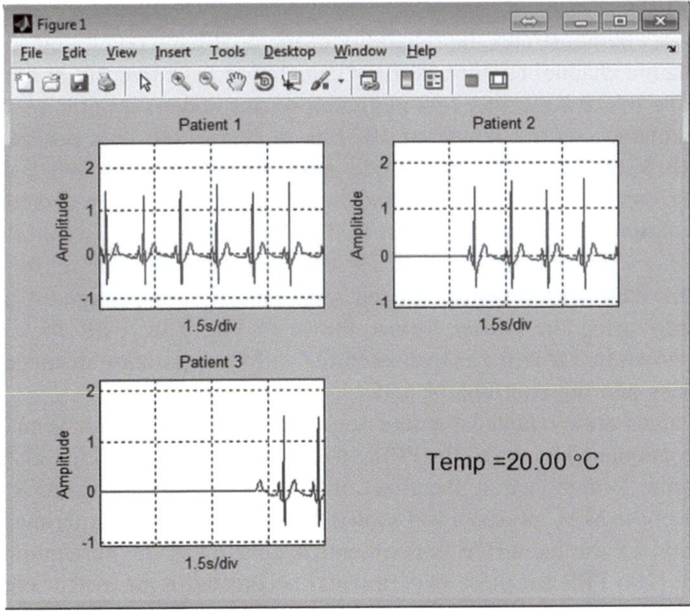

Fig. 6.10 Multi-signal monitoring implemented in Matlab

6.6 On-Body Evaluation of the Dual-Band WBAN Communication System

On-body evaluation of the dual-band communication system is performed in order to demonstrate the performance of the MAC protocol under on-body multi sensor communication scenarios. Multiple communication scenarios shown in Table 6.1 are developed based on the positioning of sensor nodes and coordinator node.

Network performance parameters, such as BER, sensor initialization delay are experimentally evaluated for each scenario. All the experiments are carried out using four sensor nodes. Sensor nodes are initiated in a random manner during the experiments. All the sensor nodes transmit at a PRF of 100 MHz. PPB values for each sensor node are controlled by changing the width of data bits generated by the micro-controller modules of the sensor nodes. The transmit spectrums of all the sensor nodes are set to fall within the FCC regulated spectral mask. Figure 6.11 depicts shows the average UWB transmit spectrum for a sensor node used in the experiments.

6.6.1 BER Performance Analysis

BER analysis demonstrates the reliability of the dual-band communication system under dynamic channel conditions. BER calculation is carried out in the following manner. The micro-controller of a particular sensor node is programmed to send a data bit sequence with a length of 10^8 bits in segmented data packets. This bit sequence is known to both sensor node and coordinator node. When the coordinator node receives data from a sensor node, it transfers the received data to a Matlab program that calculates the BER. The Matlab program uses all the bits in a data packet except the *Sync* portion for BER calculation. Four sensor nodes are used in the BER experiments. All the sensor nodes are configured to transmit continuously using the packet format shown in Fig. 6.1a. BER for a particular scenario shown in Table 6.1 is evaluated for various separation distances between sensor nodes and the coordinator node.

BER values are evaluated for four scenarios. In the first three scenarios, BER values are calculated by fixing the PPB values of each sensor node to 20, 50 and 100 PPBs in order to demonstrate the effect of PPB on BER. Dynamic BER allocation procedure of the MAC protocol is disabled for these fixed PPB experiments. Sensor initialization for the fixed PPB experiments is done using the maximum allowable PPB value (100 PPB for these experiments) according to the sensor node initialization procedure described in Chap. 3. After initialization, sensor nodes go back to sending data using the fixed PPB values assigned to each sensor node. A fourth experiment is carried out in order to evaluate the BER when the dynamic BER allocation procedure of the MAC protocol is enabled. Coordinator node assigns a PPB value range from 20 to 100 PPB according to the procedure described in Chap. 3 in an attempt to keep the BER threshold for each sensor node at 10^{-4} or the closest

Table 6.1 Different communication scenarios

Scenario name	Number of users	Coordinator position	Sensor node position	Body moments
Scenario 1	1	Off-body	On-body	Still
Scenario 2	1	Off-body	On-body	Walking
Scenario 3	1	On-body	On-body	Walking
Scenario 4	2	Off-body	On-body	Still

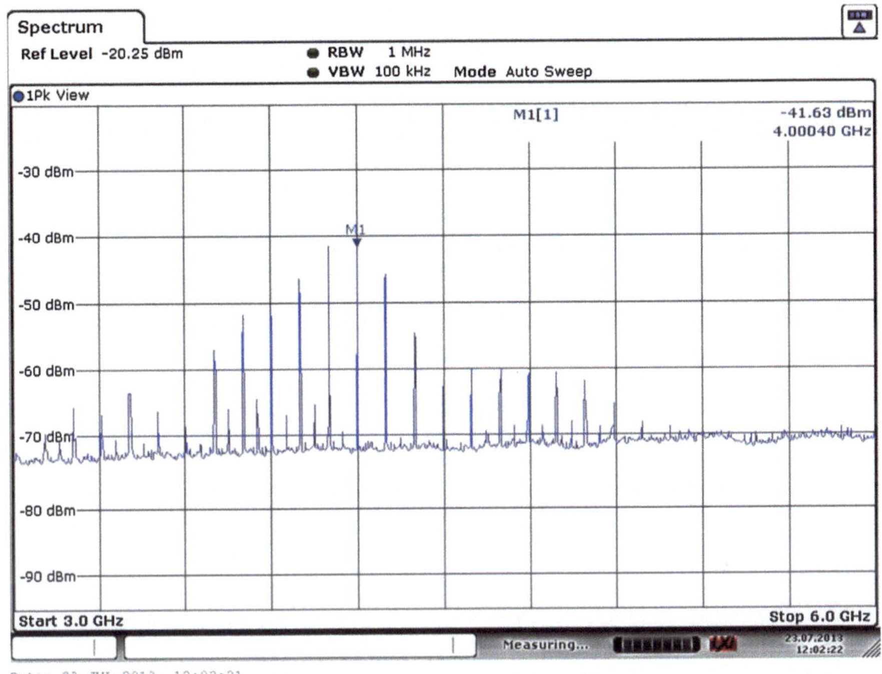

Fig. 6.11 Measured average transmit power spectrum at 100 MHz PRF

possible value. Fixed PPB experiments are used as control experiments that highlight the performance improvement introduced by the dynamic BER allocation procedure. All the experiments are carried out in a normal laboratory set up in order to simulate an indoor propagation environment. It should be noted that the receive signal strength at a given distance from a sensor nodes are largely dependent on the antenna properties such as directivity and gain.[1]

---

[1] These experiments were carried out using the antennas that were developed in house and available at the moment of the experiments. Link budget shown in Chap. 5 gives a rough estimate for the range of the UWB link.

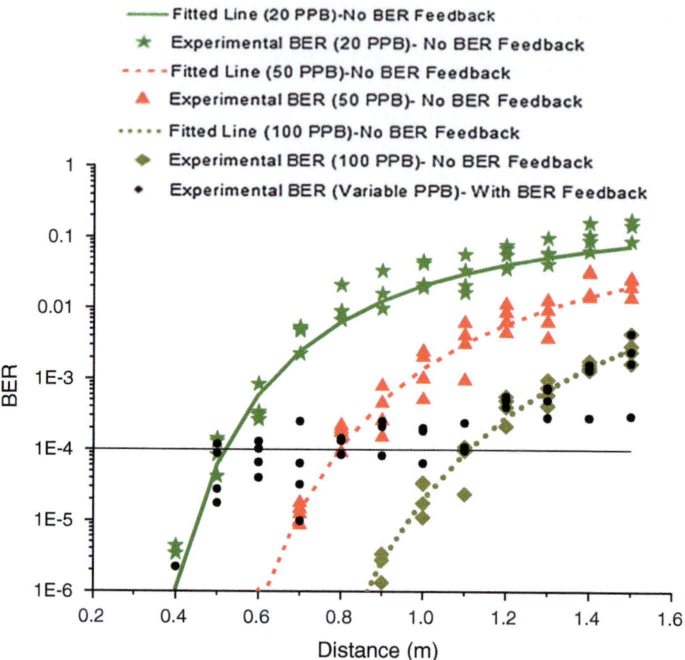

Fig. 6.12 Experimental BER variations with distance for *Scenario 1*

6.6.1.1 BER Analysis for Scenario 1

Figure 6.12 depicts the BER variation for *Scenario 1*. In this scenario, data communication occurs between four on-body sensor nodes and a coordinator node placed away from the body. All four sensor nodes are attached to a single user in a similar experimental setup to that shown in Fig. 6.9. Each point in Fig. 6.12 represents a BER value recorded for a particular sensor node at a certain distance away from the coordinator node. Distance between the user's body and the receiving antenna of the coordinator node is considered as the separation distance for this experiment. User's body is kept still throughout the BER evaluation period. BER values recorded by all four sensor nodes for various separation distances are plotted in Fig. 6.12. BER evaluation is carried out three times for a particular distance, and the average BER is plotted for each sensor node.

It can be seen from Fig. 6.12 that the recorded BER values follow a logarithmic decay. Four sensor nodes used in this experiment recorded BER values with a slight variation from each other for the same separation distance. These variations occur mainly due to different orientations of the UWB transmit antennas. Different antenna orientations cause UWB signals to propagate in different paths towards the receiving antenna at the coordinator. Fading characteristics and multi-path characteristics of these propagations paths differ from each other causing different BER values for each sensor node.

Fixed BER experiments demonstrate that the BER for a certain distance depends on the PPB value of a particular data transmission. A higher PPB transmission results in a lower BER than a lower PPB transmission for the same separation distance. These experimental results confirm the analytical BER results obtained in Chap. 3 for a short range UWB based WBAN.

Above-mentioned property of multiple PPB UWB transmission is utilized in order to keep the BER at a constant value of 10^{-4} in the variable PPB experiment where BER compensation procedure of the MAC protocol is enabled. Results in Fig. 6.12 show that BER values for the variable PPB experiment stay close to the 10^{-4} value for separation distance range of 0.5 m to 1.1 m. BER values for separation distances lower than 0.5 m stay below the 10^{-4} line following the BER trend line for 20 PPB transmission while BER values for separation distances above 1.1 m follow the BER trend line for 100 PPB transmission. This is caused by the restriction in the MAC protocol that limits the minimum PPB value to 20 and the maximum PPB value to 100. For separation distances between 0.5 and1.1 m, the MAC protocol dynamically varies the PPB value such that it is kept at a closest possible value to 10^{-4}. This result shows that the dynamic PPB scheme presented in this chapter can be used as a mechanism to improve the performance of a UWB communication system in terms of BER for WBAN applications. Figure 6.12 also depicts the fitted trend lines for each of the fixed PPB experiments. These fitted lines are used in the BER plots for other communication scenarios as guide lines in order to compare the BER results of a particular scenario with that of *Scenario 1*.

6.6.1.2 BER Analysis for Scenario 2

BER results shown in Fig. 6.13 for *Scenario 2* demonstrate the BER performance of the communication system when the user is engaged in walking at normal speed. For a fair assessment of the BER at each distance, user is made to walk in concentric circles that are at various distances from the coordinator node such that the sensor node antennas are facing towards the coordinator node all the time. Distance from the UWB receiving antenna to the user's body is considered as the separation distance in this experiment. It can be observed that the BER recorded for fixed PPB experiments in this scenario are higher than that of the *Scenario 1*. This is mainly cause by the worsened channel conditions due to high signal dispersion, increased reflections and diffractions of the UWB signals, and increased attenuation due to absorption of the electromagnetic signals by human body parts that interact with the signal propagation path. Furthermore, it can be seen from Fig. 6.13 that the BER values for sensor nodes that are at same separation distance from the coordinator node show a larger variation compared with that in *Scenario 1*. This is mainly due to different effects of complex body motions on different sensor nodes that are placed at various positions on the upper body. Variable PPB experiment conducted under this scenario demonstrates the BER improvement introduced by the BER compensation procedure under dynamic

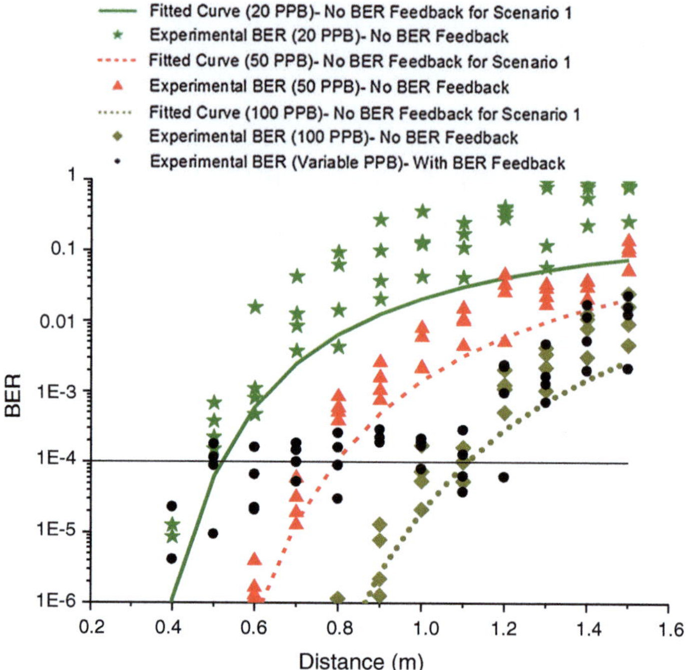

Fig. 6.13 Experimental BER variations for *Scenario 2*

channel conditions. It should be noted that BER is marked as '*1*' for instances where it is not possible to decode any bits during the experiments.

6.6.1.3 BER Analysis for Scenario 3

Scenario 3 represents experiments carried out by placing both transmitter and receiver UWB antennas on user's body as shown in Fig. 6.14. Positions of the sensor nodes are fixed while position of the receiver UWB antenna is changed from user's chest area to upper part of user's left leg. Average distance between sensor and coordinator UWB antennas are taken as the separation distance for this experiment. User is made to walk at normal speeds during the BER evaluation period. Figure 6.15 depicts the BER variation for this scenario. It should be noted that only the BER values for 20 and 50 PPB fixed PPB experiments are plotted in Fig. 6.15 since only these experiments resulted in a considerable BER value for this distance range. Results show a degraded BER performance compared that of *Scenario 1*. This is mainly caused by the degrations in signal conditions due to the increased reflections and diffractions caused by complex body motions and irregular geometry of the human body. Increased attenuation due to the absorption of UWB signals from human skin and garment materials also degrades the BER

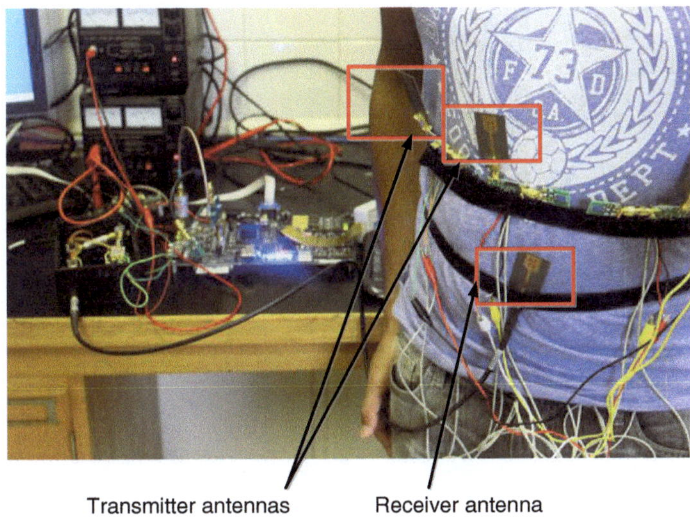

Fig. 6.14 Experimental set up for on-body measurements

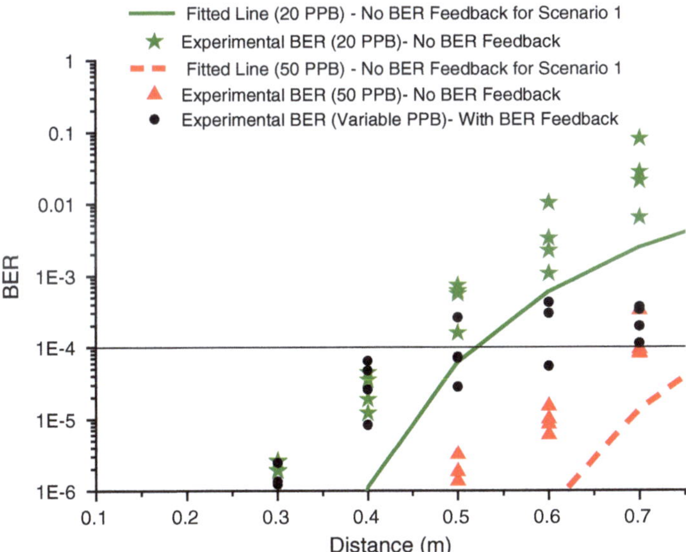

Fig. 6.15 Experimental BER variations for *Scenario 3*

performance of the system. Furthermore, results for the variable PPB experiments demonstrates the improvements of the BER for on-body communication channels that can be achieved using the BER compensation procedure.

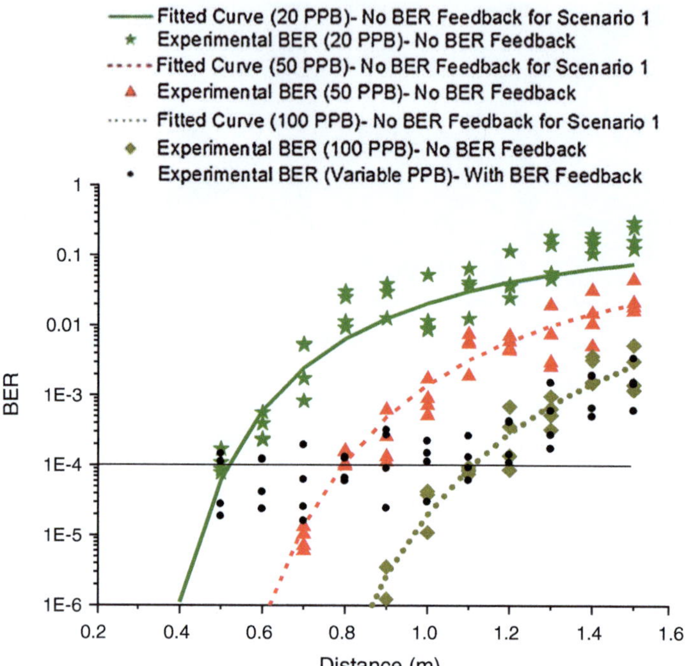

Fig. 6.16 Experimental BER variation of *Scenario 4*

6.6.1.4 BER Analysis for Scenario 4

Scenario 4 follows the same experimental procedure as in *Scenario 1* except for the fact that sensor nodes are placed on two users such that each user carries two on-body sensor nodes. Both users are placed at equal distances from coordinator node. Figure 6.16 presents the BER variation for different separation distances. BER variation for this experiment behaves in a similar pattern to that of *Scenario 1*. The scheduled nature of the data transmission in dual-band MAC protocol helps to avoid data collisions between sensor nodes that belong to the same user as well as sensor nodes that belong to different users. Hence, BER for both *Scenario 1* and *Scenario 2* show similar behavior.

6.6.2 Initialization Delay of Sensor Nodes

Sensor initialization delay represents the time taken for a sensor node to register in the communication system and starts data communication. A sensor node goes through the procedure shown in Fig. 6.17 during a sensor initialization stage. This sensor initialization procedure is further described under Chap. 3. During the

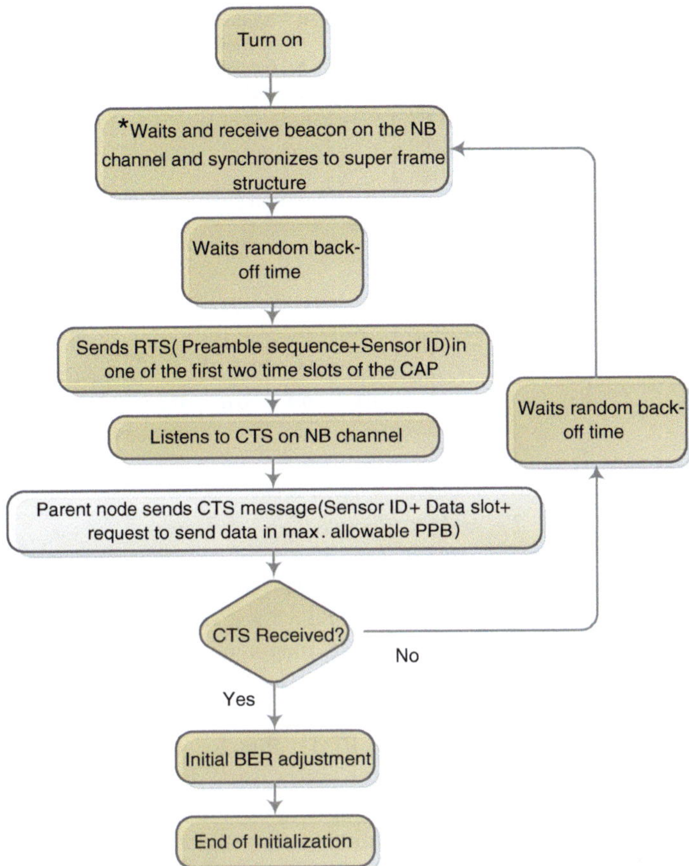

Fig. 6.17 Sensor initialization procedure

sensor initialization, a sensor node uses the maximum allowable PPB value (100 PPB for this experiment) in order to transmit a Ready To Send (RTS) message. After receiving a Clear To Send (CTS) message, a sensor node goes through a BER compensation period where sensor node and coordinator node negotiate a final PPB value to be used for that particular instance in order to transmit at a minimum possible PPB value while keeping the BER below or equal to 10^{-4}. Initialization delay depends on many parameters, such as BER of the system at a particular instance, congestion in the initialization slots of the super frame structure and propagation delay of the wireless signals. For this experiment initialization delay is measured from the time a sensor node receives the first beacon until the time where the sensor node start data transmission. All the sensor nodes are turned on at the same time. Initialization delay for a particular sensor node can be expressed using the following equation.

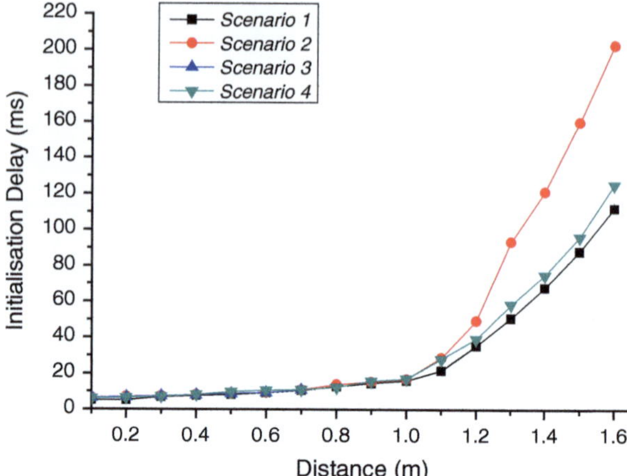

Fig. 6.18 Experimental variation of sensor initialization delay with distance for different communication scenarios

$$T_{ID} = N \times (T_{RTS} + T_{CTS}) + T_{BER} \tag{6.1}$$

where T_{ID} is the sensor initialization delay, T_{RTS} is the time difference between a beacon reception and transmission of an RTS by a sensor node, T_{CTS} is the time difference between transmission of an RTS message and successful reception of a CTS message or maximum time-out time in case of an unsuccessful CTS reception by a sensor node, $N = 1, 2, 3 \ldots 10$ is the number of initialization attempts and T_{BER} is the time taken to negotiate a final PPB value for data transmission. Sensor initialization delay is measured at sensor nodes using a timer to measure the time difference between the reception of the first beacon message and successful initialization of the sensor. This information is then transferred to a computer terminal at the end of initialization using a data packet. Figure 6.18 depicts the variation of average sensor initialization delay with distance for the variable PPB experiments in different scenarios shown in Table 6.1. Average initialization delay is calculated by averaging the initialization delay recorded by all four sensors over three experiments conducted for each separation distance.

It can be seen from Fig. 6.18 that the initialization delay increases with the separation distance in general. This variation can be explained by the increase of BER and propagation delay with increasing separation distance. High BER values cause the initialization request messages to be erroneous, which results in increased number of initialization attempts. However, sensor initialization delay for all the scenarios showed only a little variation from each other up to a distance of 1.1 m. This is due to the fact that all the initialization messages use the maximum allowable PPB value of 100 PPB for sensor initialization. Hence, the effect of BER on initialization delay affects equally for all the scenarios within this separation distance. A rapid increase in initialization delay can be observed above a separation distance of 1.1 m; after which BER can no longer be contained closer to 10^{-4} due to the maximum PPB limitation of 100 PPB. *Scenario 2* showed the highest deviation in initialization delay above the separation distance of 1.1 m.

This is mainly due to higher BER of *Scenario 2* compared to other scenarios over this separation distance range. These results further highlight the importance of the multiple PPB scheme in order to keep the sensor initialization delay at an acceptable level.

6.7 Power Consumption of Dual-Band Sensor Nodes in WBAN Operation

Power consumption is one of the important areas for battery powered WBAN applications. Both wearable and implantable WBAN sensor nodes should be able to operate with minimum intervention for longer periods. UWB transmitters are inherently low power consuming compared to UWB receivers mainly due to its low complexity circuit design. The sensor platform presented in Chap. 5 avoids the high complexity and power hungry UWB receiver by using a narrowband receiver. Even further improvements in power consumption can be achieved by proper design of the MAC protocol.

One of the main attributes of the MAC protocol design presented in this chapter is that it uses the minimum PPB value that is achievable at a given time in order to transmit data while maintaining the BER approximately at 10^{-4}. Using the minimum PPB value for data transmission ensures that the duration of UWB data transmission is kept at its optimum value throughout the data transmission cycle. Duration of data transmission is one of the key factors that determine the energy consumption of a MAC protocol. Hence, keeping the duration of data transmission slot to an optimum value helps to optimize the power consumption of sensor nodes.

The experimental setup shown in Fig. 6.19 is used in order to measure the overall current consumption of the sensor nodes. A probe with low capacitance is used for voltage measurement across the 10 Ω resistor and all the higher order bypass capacitors are removed from sensor nodes in order to minimize the capacitive effects on the measured waveforms.

Figure 6.20 depicts the overall current consumption of a periodic sensor node that transmits at 100 PPB with a packet length of 50 bits and two continuous sensor nodes that transmit at 20 and 100 PPB with a packet length of 100 bits. All the sensor nodes transmit at a PRF of 100 MHz. Current consumption measurements have been carried out over a period of 2 ms (i.e. two super frame durations). Figure 6.20 also shows current consumption for different stages of a sensor start-up period. Sensor nodes are programmed to send data packets with dummy pay-load after the first beacon reception for the purpose of demonstrating the variation of current consumption during a data communication period of the dual MAC protocol. Narrowband receiver is continuously operated throughout the data communication period for continuous sensor nodes in order to receive control packets from the coordinator node. Periodic sensor nodes go into sleep mode

Fig. 6.19 Current measurement test set up

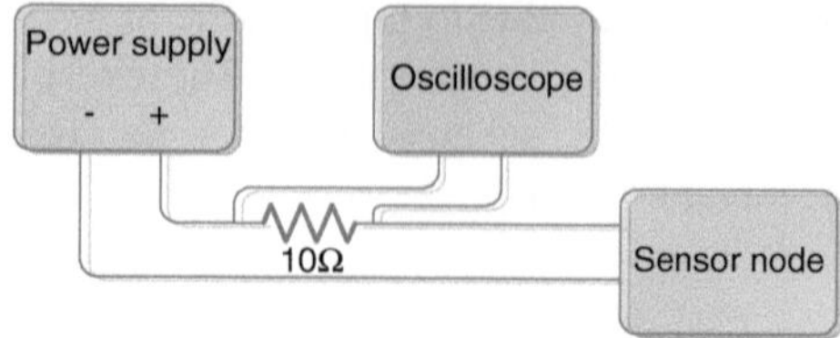

operation after receiving the acknowledgement packet for the data packet that is transmitted during the super frame time slot.

It can be seen from the results that all the data communication scenarios consume a peak current of approximately 16.5 mA. Sleep mode current consumption for periodic sensor nodes is observed to be 0.3 mA. UWB transmission consumes the most amount of current during a data communication cycle. Current consumption of the UWB transmitter is mostly affected by the operation of high frequency Voltage Controlled Oscillator (VCO) in the RF portion of the circuit. However, due to the high data rate of UWB transmission, duration of data transmission occupies only a small percentage of the super frame duration resulting in low energy consumption. This presents a unique advantage of the UWB technology over other technologies in terms of energy saving. Periodic sensor nodes largely benefit from this duty-cycled transmission since a large amount of data can be accumulated over a long time before sending at a high data rate. Furthermore, dual-band MAC protocol ensures that UWB sensor nodes are transmitting at the optimum PPB value for a given distance. For example, UWB transmitter of a particular continuous sensor node located at a separation distance of 0.2 m transmits data at 20 PPB rather than transmitting at the maximum allowable value of 100 PPB. This results in an energy saving of approximately 5 % for that particular distance. This energy saving increases to a large value over the long life cycle of a WBAN sensor node. Use of a narrowband receiver further enhances the power savings of a dual-band sensor node. An equivalent UWB receiver has a power consumption that is several times larger than a narrowband receiver [11–13]. Hence, use of a narrowband receiver in the sensor node presented in Chap. 5 increases its lifetime by several times.

Table 6.2 depicts the average power and energy consumption of major sections of the sensor node that are related to data communication scenarios shown in Fig. 6.20. Power is averaged over one transmission cycle. For example, transmission cycle for a continuous sensor node is considered to be the duration of one super frame (1 ms) and transmission cycle for a period sensor node is considered to be the duration between two consecutive transmissions (10 s for this particular experiment). Table 6.2 also show the energy consumption per useful data bit transmitted using the UWB transmitter that can be obtained using (6.2).

$$E_{bit}\left(\frac{J}{bit}\right) = \left(\frac{I_{TX}(A) \times V_s(V) \times T_{TX}(s)}{B_{TX}}\right) \tag{6.2}$$

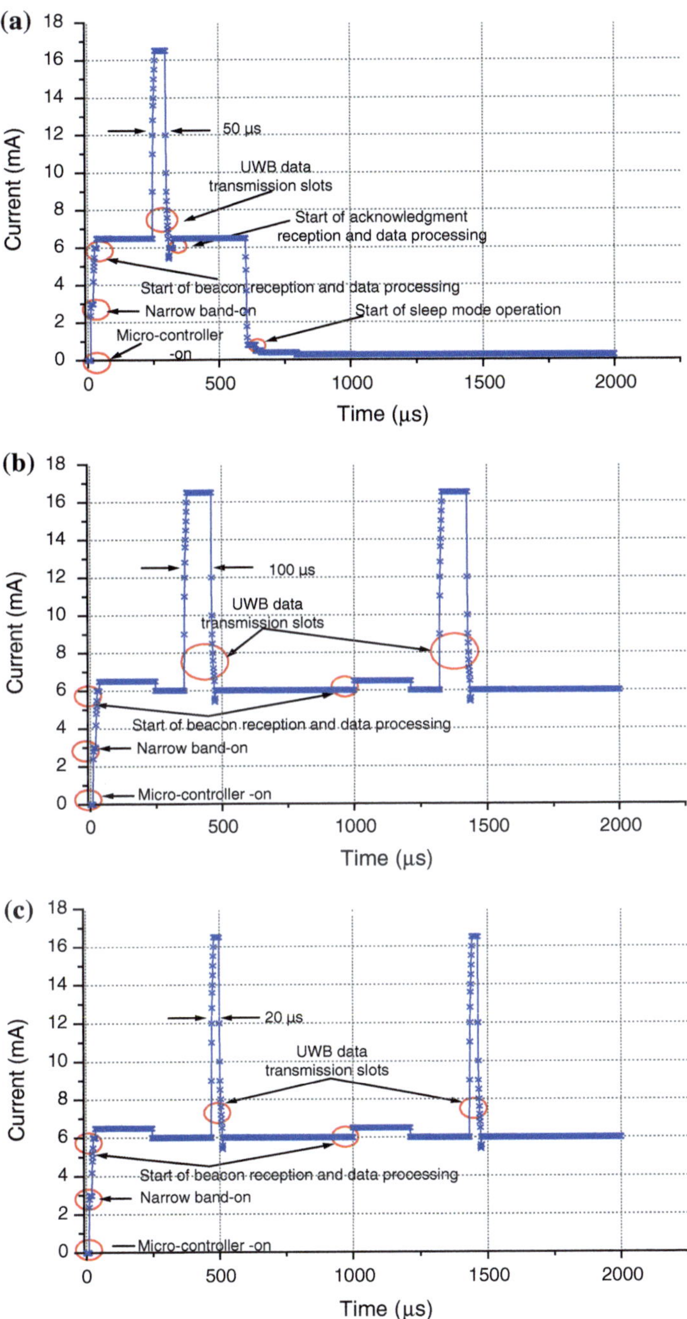

Fig. 6.20 a Current consumption of a periodic sensor node transmitting at 100 PPB, current consumption of a continuous sensor node transmitting at **b** 100 PPB, **c** 20 PPB

Table 6.2 Power and energy consumption of different data communication scenarios

| | Scenario | | |
	A	B	C
Reference	Figure 6.19a	Figure 6.19b	Figure 6.19c
UWB transmitter (mW)	0.15	3.1	0.6
Narrowband receiver (mW)	0.64	9.9	9.92
Micro-controller (mW)	0.68	10.48	10.52
Total power (mW)	1.47	23.48	21.04
Energy per useful data bit (nJ/bit)	27.22	54.45	10.89

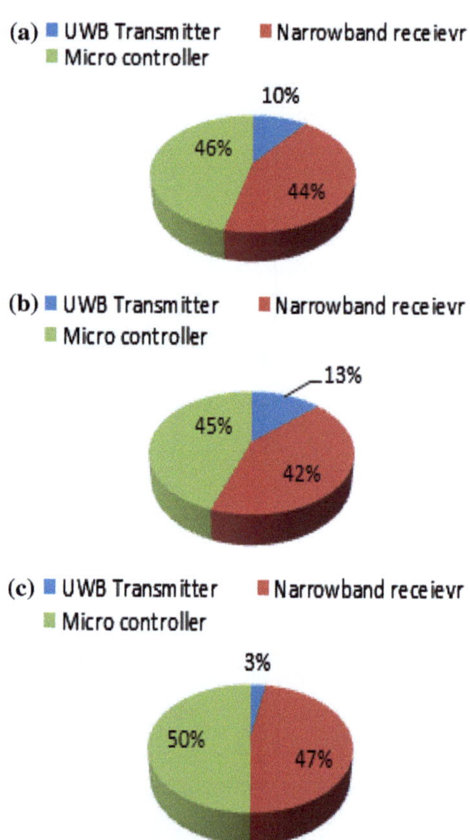

Fig. 6.21 Percentage power consumption for different components of the sensor node for three scenarios given in Table 6.2

where E_{bit} is the energy consumption per useful transmit data bit, I_{TX} is the current consumption during transmission, V_s is the supply voltage, T_{TX} is the time duration of data transmission and B_{TX} is the total number of bits that are transmitted. It should be noted that power consumption of data sensing using either the analog front-end or digital data input depends on a particular application and are not consider for this calculation. It was observed that the analog/RF front-end consumes a current of 6 mA and digital communication with the micro-controller consumes only a negligible amount of current in addition to the normal operational current of the micro-controller.

It can be observed from Table 6.2 that the micro controller consumes the largest portion of power among the main sections involved in data transmission. Power consumption of the UWB transmitter is considerably low due to its low duty cycled high data rate transmission. A similar experiment is carried out in [14] in order to investigate the power consumption of a wireless sensor node based on a 2.4 GHz transceiver module. This investigation shows much higher levels of power consumption compared to this design. Figure 6.21 demonstrates percentage power consumption for each scenario shown in Table 6.2.

6.8 Conclusion

This chapter describes the implementation of a dual-band MAC protocol and evaluation of its various performance parameters such as BER, initialization delay and power consumption. Pulse synchronization and bit synchronization play an important role in accurate detection of UWB data. The unique pulse synchronization mechanism described in this chapter avoids the requirement of an ADC with high sampling rate in order to sample narrow UWB pulses. On-body BER evaluation results presented in this chapter confirms the efficiency introduced by multiple PPB scheme for short-range WBAN communications. A MAC protocol can be designed to have dynamic allocation of the number of pulses per bit. This ensures that the sensor nodes transmit data while maintaining an acceptable BER. BER evaluation is carried out for various scenarios based on the position of the sensor nodes, number of users and presence of body motion. It can be observed from the results that the body motion adversely affects the BER performance of a WBAN communication system. A multiple PPB scheme is able to compensate for the changes in the BER levels that occur because of rapidly changing channel conditions.

The dynamic PPB scheme described in this chapter ensures that sensor nodes always transmit at the minimum PPB value while maintaining an acceptable BER level. This mechanism enables the sensor nodes to operate at optimum power consumption while maintaining a reliable data communication link. The cross layer implementation of MAC protocol, together with the dual-band hardware implementation of sensor node provides a power efficient communication system that can be used efficiently in WBAN applications that require various data transmission capabilities.

Acknowledgment The authors would like to thank Dr. Tharaka Dissanayake for his help in designing the UWB antenna used for the high frequency simulations.

References

1. H.C. Keong, M.R. Yuce, Low data rate ultra wideband ECG monitoring system, in *the IEEE Engineering in Medicine and Biology Society Conference (IEEE EMBC08)*, pp. 3413–3416, Aug 2008
2. H.C. Keong, K.M. Thotahewa, M.R. Yuce, Transmit-only ultra wide band (UWB) body sensors and collision analysis. IEEE Sens. J. **13**, 1949–1958 (2013)
3. K.M. Thotahewa, J.-M. Redoute, M.R. Yuce, Implementation of a dual band body sensor node, in *IEEE MTT-S International Microwave Workshop Series on RF and Wireless Technologies for Biomedical and Healthcare (IMWS-Bio2013)*, 2013
4. H.C. Keong, T.S.P. See, M.R. Yuce, An ultra-wideband wireless body area network: evaluation in static and dynamic channel conditions. Sens. Actuators A Phys. **180**, 137–147 (2012)
5. A. Taparugssanagorn, C. Pomalaza-Raez, R. Tesi, M. Hamalainen, J. Iinatti, Effect of body motion and the type of antenna on the measured UWB channel characteristics in medical applications of wireless body area networks, in *IEEE International Conference on Ultra-Wideband*, pp. 332–336, 2009
6. K. Thotahewa, J. Khan, M. Yuce, Power efficient ultra wide band based wireless body area networks with narrowband feedback path. IEEE Trans. Mobile Comput. pp. 1–1 (2013) (in pre-print version)
7. K.M. Silva, M.R Yuce, J.Y. Khan, Multiple access protocol for UWB wireless body area networks (WBANs) with narrowband feedback path, *in Proceedings of the IEEE International Symposium on Applied Sciences in Biomedical and Communication Technologies (ISABEL)*, 2011
8. K.M. Thotahewa, J.-M. Redoute, M.R. Yuce, A low-power, wearable, dual-band wireless body area network system: development and experimental evaluation (submitted)
9. http://www.altera.com/, 2014
10. www.mathworks.com, 2014
11. P. Jian, Z. Sheng, J. Benzhou, L. Xiaokang, Performance analysis of three kinds of non-coherent detectors for ultra-wideband communications, in *7th International Conference on Wireless Communications, Networking and Mobile Computing*, pp. 1–4, 2011
12. Y. Gao, Y. Zheng, S. Diao, W. Toh, C. Ang, M. Je, C. Heng, Low-power ultra-wideband wireless telemetry transceiver for medical sensor applications. IEEE Trans. Biomed. Eng. **58**(3), 768–772 (2011)
13. D. Barras, R. Meyer-Piening, G. von Bueren, W. Hirt, H. Jaeckel, A low-power baseband ASIC for an energy-collection IR-UWB receiver. IEEE J. Solid-State Circuits **44**, 1721–1733 (2009)
14. S. Wang, R. O'Keeffe, N. Wang, M. Hayes, B. O'Flynn, S.C. Ó Mathúna, Practical wireless sensor networks power consumption metrics for building energy management applications, in *23rd European Conference on Construction Informatics, Cork, Ireland*, 12–14 Sept 2011

Chapter 7
Electromagnetic Effects of IR-UWB Implant Communication

Abstract With the increased use of Impulse Radio-Ultra-Wideband (IR-UWB) devices within or at close proximity to the human body, it is of utmost importance to analyze the electromagnetic effects caused by those devices. As human tissue is exposed to the electromagnetic signals emitted from IR-UWB devices, they absorb a certain amount of transmitted power and convert it into heat. This phenomenon causes a temperature increase in the human tissue. The heating effect of the human tissue is significant for high-frequency and high-bandwidth signals, such as the IR-UWB signals. The temperature increase of the tissue material should be regulated in order to prevent any adverse effects caused by the exposure to electromagnetic signals. Specific Absorption Rate (SAR) and Specific Absorption (SA) provide a good indication of the amount of power absorbed by the himan tissues. This chapter presents the SAR, SA and temperature variation of the human body caused by IR-UWB signals. An IR-UWB based Wireless Capsule Endoscopy (WCE) that operates inside the human abdomen is used as the main application for this study. This analysis compares the compliance of the IR-UWB based WCE devices with international safety regulations. A voxel model of the human body consisting of human tissue simulating materials is used for this simulation-based study. The tissue properties, such as relative permittivity, are characterized according to the incident signal frequency and age of the tissue sample during simulations. The SAR and SA variations are analyzed using the Finite Integration Technique (FIT) as the discretization model.

Keywords SAR/SA · Wireless capsule endoscopy · Head implant · Electro-magnetic effects · Temperature increase · Bio-heat equation · IR-UWB

7.1 Introduction

Wireless communication for implantable sensor devices has drawn the attention of researchers in recent years due to the several advantages it possesses, such as minimizing restrictions in daily activities, facilitating less invasive surgical

K. M. S. Thotahewa et al., *Ultra Wideband Wireless Body Area Networks*,
DOI: 10.1007/978-3-319-05287-8_7,
© Springer International Publishing Switzerland 2014

procedures and offering remote control and monitoring [1–4]. With the extensive use of wireless devices within or at close proximity to the human body, electromagnetic effects caused by the interaction between radio frequency waves and human tissues are of paramount importance. SAR, which determines the amount of signal energy absorbed by the human body tissue, is used as the index for many standards to regulate the amount of exposure of the human body to electromagnetic radiation [5, 6]. Various regulatory bodies provide different assessment methods and different maximum allowable SAR limits for the human tissue that are exposed to electromagnetic signals. Regulations by the International Council on Non-Ionizing Radiation Protection (ICNIRP) standard limit the localized 10 g averaged SAR in the head to 2 W/kg for signals in the range of 10 kHz to 10 GHz [5]. The IEEE/ICES C95.1-2005 standard limits the 10 g averaged SAR value over a six minute time period to 1.6 W/kg [6]. Additional regulations are applied for pulsed transmission schemes in order to prevent auditory effects. A 2 mJ/kg SA averaged over 10 g tissue weight for a single pulse is applied by the ICNIRP standard while 576 J/kg averaged over a 10 g tissue for a six minute period is applied by the IEEE/ICES C95.1-2005 standard. Some of the international standards that provide regulations on SAR limits are depicted in Table 7.1.

Studies have shown that a temperature increase in excess of 1 °C can prove harmful to the human body [5]. Many studies have been carried out in order to assess the effect of radio frequency signals [7–15]. Most of the research work in this area has been done based on on-body scenarios, where most of the signal propagation occurs through air interface before coming into contact with the body tissues [10–15]. Because of the increased use of implantable wireless devices, where most of the electromagnetic wave propagation occurs within the human tissue, it is important to analyze the effects of those devices on the human body. Only a few studies found in the literature investigate the effects of in-body propagation of electromagnetic waves on human tissue [7, 8]. With the emergence of new techniques to record physiological data such as neural recording systems [16, 17] and WCE [18], the need for high data rate wireless transmission has become a key requirement for implantable devices. Impulse Radio Ultra Wide Band (IR-UWB) can be identified as a technology that caters the need for high data rate while requiring low power consumption.

As UWB communication becomes more prominent in high data rate implant communication [16–18, 20, 21], it is important to investigate the electromagnetic effects caused by a UWB transmitter implanted in the human body. Several publications are found in the literature that have analysed the effect of UWB on the human body based on on-body scenarios [12–15]. They investigate the SAR variation caused by a UWB transmitting source placed externally at a close proximity of the human body. These results provide a general understanding about the electromagnetic effects caused by on-body propagation of UWB signals. Many reported studies used homogeneous human body models without considering the differences in properties of various types of tissue materials, which can significantly affect the results. SAR variation also depends on antenna properties, such as directivity, orientation and gain. A few reported studies demonstrate the effects of

Table. 7.1 Electromagnetic exposure limits provided by various regulatory bodies [19]

	Standard	Averaging method	Freq. range	Whole body avg. SAR (W kg^{-1})	Localised SAR (head and trunk) (W kg^{-1})	Limbs (W kg^{-1})
Occupational exposure/ controlled environment	ICNIRP 2009	Averaged over cross section of 1 cm^2 perpendicular to current direction and for 6 min period	100 kHz–10 GHz	0.4	10	20
	IEEE/ICES C95.1-2005	Averaged over 10 g tissue for 6 min	100 kHz–3 GHz	0.4	10	20
	Health Canada Safety Code 6 2009	Tissue volume in form of cube and averaged over 6 min period	100 kHz–6 GHz	0.4	8	20
	CENELEC 1995	Averaged over 10 g tissue for 6 min	10 kHz–30 GHz	0.4	10	20
General public exposure/ controlled environment	ICNIRP 2009	Averaged over cross section of 1 cm^2 perpendicular to current direction and for 6 min period	100 kHz–10 GHz	0.08	2	4
	IEEE/ICES C95.1-2005	Averaged over 10 g tissue in a cube and averaged over 30 min period	100 kHz–3 GHz	2	2	4
	Health Canada Safety Code 6 2009	Tissue volume in form of cube	100 kHz–6 GHz	0.08	1.6	4
	CENELEC 1995	Averaged over 10 g tissue for 6 min	10 kHz–30 GHz	0.08	2	4

radio frequency transmission from implantable devices inside the human body [7, 8, 22]. Some of them report the SAR variations caused by implantable devices operating at low frequency bands such as MICS and ISM bands [7, 8]. The work reported in [22] illustrates the SAR variation caused by an IR-UWB source inside the human stomach. The latter uses the Finite Difference Time Domain (FDTD) computation method, which discretises the derivatives in Maxwell's curl equations [23] using finite differences. However, [22] has not considered an antenna model in the simulations; additionally, the FCC regulations that govern the UWB indoor propagation are not taken into account. Many studies have analysed path-loss as the sole indicator of electromagnetic power absorption [24–27]. However, SAR and SA measurements can be associated easily with the temperature increase in the human tissue.

This chapter presents the electromagnetic effects and thermal effects of IR-UWB implant communication, which are important safety measures in the applications of body area network applications. IR-UWB based WCE is used as the application of focus in this chapter. A human anatomical body model developed by CST Studio [28], which has been recognised by the Federal Communications Commission (FCC) [29] as a suitable simulation tool for SAR calculations, is used to simulate the human tissue properties at UWB frequencies. An implantable antenna working at UWB frequencies is used as the source of the UWB signals. The 4-Cole Cole model [30] is used in order to consider the dispersive nature of the tissue materials at these high frequencies. In addition, the effect of the human age is considered when calculating the tissue properties such as relative permittivity. An IR-UWB pulse operating at a centre frequency of 4 GHz and a bandwidth of 1 GHz has been chosen as the excitation to the antenna. This range is selected so that the UWB spectrum has minimum interference from other wireless technologies, such as 5 GHz Wi-Fi.

7.2 Simulation Models and Methods

This section givens a brief introduction to the simulation models and methods used for calculation of SAR and temperature increase of human tissue that is exposed to IR-UWB signals.

7.2.1 Effect of Human Tissue Properties on SAR

A compilation of experimental and theoretical results on human tissue property variation depending on the incident frequency provided in [30, 31] proves that the former behaves differently at different incident frequencies. This is due to a property known as dielectric dispersion. The SAR value for a certain material subjected to an electromagnetic field can be calculated by (7.1) [32].

$$\text{SAR} = \frac{1}{2}\frac{\sigma}{\rho}|\mathbf{E}|^2 \tag{7.1}$$

where E is the root mean square (RMS) electric field strength, ρ is the mass density (in kg/m^3), and σ is the conductivity of the tissue. The electric field and the magnetic field in the frequency domain can be described by Maxwell's curl equations in the frequency domain as below:

$$\nabla \times \mathbf{E}(\omega) = -j\omega\mu\mathbf{H}(\omega) \tag{7.2}$$

$$\nabla \times \mathbf{H}(\omega) = j\omega\varepsilon_0\varepsilon_r'(\omega)\mathbf{E}(\omega) \tag{7.3}$$

where $j = \sqrt{-1}$ is the imaginary unit, ω is the angular frequency, $\mathbf{E}(\omega)$ and $\mathbf{H}(\omega)$ are time-harmonic electric and magnetic fields, μ is the permeability, ε_0 is the free space permittivity and $\varepsilon_r'(\omega)$ is the frequency dependent complex relative permittivity. Because of the dependency of the electric field on $\varepsilon_r'(\omega)$, the SAR variation inherently depends on the relative permittivity of the material, which itself depends on the incident frequency of the electromagnetic signal. The behavior of the complex relative permittivity for different tissue types differs from each other, especially at higher frequency ranges such as UWB. Hence, it is not advised to use straightforward homogeneous body models to simulate the electromagnetic effects at higher frequencies. The simulations presented in this chapter use the CST Studio voxel human model, which is a human body model consisting of a mixture of tissue materials such as brain, bone, intestinal tissue, colon tissue, fat and skin. It also considers blood flow for thermal calculations.

The frequency dependent dielectric permittivity of human tissue can be expressed as [33]:

$$\varepsilon_r'(\omega) = \varepsilon' - j\varepsilon'' = \varepsilon' - j\frac{\sigma}{\varepsilon_0\omega} = \varepsilon'\left(1 - j\frac{1}{\omega\tau}\right) \tag{7.4}$$

where ε' is the relative permittivity of the tissue material, ε'' is the out of phase loss factor, which can be expressed as $\varepsilon' = \frac{\sigma}{\varepsilon_0\omega}$ and $\tau = \frac{\varepsilon_0\varepsilon'}{\sigma}$ is the relaxation time constant. In the expression for ε'', σ represents the total conductivity of the material, which might be partially attributed by frequency dependent ionic conductivity σ_i, $\varepsilon_0 = 8.85 \times 10^{-12}$ F/m is the permittivity of the free space and ω is the angular frequency. Based on this equation, Gabriel et al. have proposed a method of evaluating the frequency dependent relative permittivity of a material by so-called 4-Cole Cole model approximation given in the equation below [30]:

$$\varepsilon_r'(\omega) = \varepsilon_\infty + \sum_{n=1}^{4}\frac{\Delta\varepsilon_n}{1 + (j\omega\tau_n)^{1-\alpha_n}} + \frac{\sigma_i}{j\omega\varepsilon_0} \tag{7.5}$$

where ε_∞ is the permittivity when $\omega \to \infty$ (permittivity in Terahertz frequencies in practical scenarios), $\Delta\varepsilon_n$ is the change in the permittivity in a specified frequency range during nth iteration, τ_n is the relaxation time during the nth iteration, α_n is the nth iteration of the distribution parameter which is a measure of the broadening of dispersion and σ_i is the static ionic conductivity. Due to the high computational complexity involved when calculating the SAR in the time domain, for example when using the FDTD method, most of the literature available for SAR variation in body tissues used an approximation method such as the Debye approximation [9] or the so called $4 \times$ L Cole Cole approximation [22] instead of the more accurate 4-Cole Cole model of tissue properties. This is mainly due to the fact that obtaining a time domain expression for $\varepsilon_r'(\omega)$ for $0 < \alpha_n < 1$ is computationally intensive. The approach followed in this chapter has been to compute the SAR in the frequency domain, which enables to use the more accurate 4-Cole Cole approximation in the obtained calculations.

Apart from the frequency dependent dispersive nature of the tissue materials, the human age affects the electromagnetic behavior of body tissues. This is mainly due to the change in the water content of tissue with age [34, 35]. Methods presented in [36] follow the Lichtenecker's exponential law for the complex permittivity based on the water content of the human tissue materials [37]. According to the information given in [37], the relative permittivity of any tissue material (i.e. real part of the complex relative permittivity (ε' in (7.4)) can be calculated as:

$$\varepsilon' = \varepsilon_w^\beta \varepsilon_t^{1-\beta} \tag{7.6}$$

where ε_W is the permittivity of water, ε_t is the age independent relative permittivity of the tissue organic material and β is the hydrate rate for the tissue material. β can be expressed as $\beta = \rho \cdot TBW$, where $TBW = 784 - 241 \cdot e^{\left\{ -\left[\frac{\ln\left(\frac{AGE}{55}\right)}{6.9589}\right]^2 \right\}}$ is the total body water index ("AGE" is the age of the tissues sample in years) [36, 38]. After some primary operations, the frequency dependent complex permittivity for body tissues can be expressed as follows [36]:

$$\varepsilon_r'(\omega) = \varepsilon_w^{\frac{\beta-\beta_A}{1-\beta_A}} \varepsilon_A^{\frac{1-\beta}{1-\beta_A}} \left(1 - j\frac{1}{\omega\tau} \right) \tag{7.7}$$

where ε_A is the age dependent relative permittivity of a reference adult tissue material which can be expressed as $\varepsilon_A = \varepsilon_w^{\beta_A} \varepsilon_t^{1-\beta_A}$ by replacing $\varepsilon' = \varepsilon_A$ in (7.6) (for present simulations, the tissue parameters of a 55 year old adult are used as reference) and β_A is the hydrate rate for adult tissues (all other parameters are described in (7.4) and (7.6)). By using the 4-Cole Cole approximation in combination with the age related tissue parameter approximations it is possible to characterize the human tissue properties with sufficient precision. This approach has been utilized in the present study. This study also considers the relative

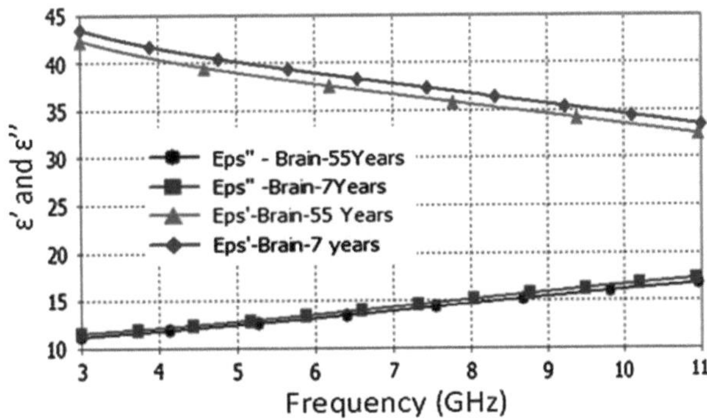

Fig. 7.1 Simulated variation of ε' and ε'' in the UWB frequency range, IEEE copyright [39]

permittivity variation of water depending on the incident frequency instead of the constant value used in [36] for age related calculations. Figure 7.1 depicts an example for the variation of ε' and ε'' as a function of frequency for the brain tissue material of a child of 7 years and a male of 55 years [39]. The basic set of tissue parameters required for the calculation (e.g. $\tau_1 - \tau_4$, $\Delta\varepsilon_1 - \Delta\varepsilon_4$ and $\alpha_1 - \alpha_4$) of the 4-Cole Cole approximation is taken from [33]. It should be observed that while ε' depends on the variation of the tissue water content with age, ε'' is largely age independent as the latter is determined by the conductivity (σ). This can be seen in Fig. 7.1.

7.2.2 SAR Calculation Method

The Finite Integration Technique (FIT) is used as the volume discretization approach for the described simulations. This technique is used to calculate the absorption loss of the body tissues by discretising the Maxwell's curl equations in a specified domain. The discretising volume element is chosen to be cubic, and appropriate boundary conditions are applied in order to define the power absorbed within that cube. Further information on the FIT model can be found in [40, 41].

SAR is defined as the power absorbed by the mass contained within that discretised volume element as shown in (7.8) [42].

$$SAR = \frac{d\left(\frac{\Delta W}{\rho dV}\right)}{dt} \tag{7.8}$$

where ΔW is the power absorbed by the discretised volume element, ρ is the density of the human tissue material, dt is the incremental time and dV is its incremental volume. Present simulations use an IR-UWB signal pulse as the excitation signal, and are conducted in order to calculate the 10 g averaged SAR so as to compare it with the ICNIRP specifications for pulse transmission [5]. The maximum SAR within the 10 g of tissue averaging volume is taken into consideration in order to demonstrate the worst-case scenario. The Specific Absorption (SA) per pulse, which is being used to introduce additional limitations for pulsed transmissions in the ICNIRP limitations, is computed using:

$$SA = SAR \times T_p \tag{7.9}$$

where T_p is the pulse duration.

It should be noted that heat sources such as the electronic components used in the implanted circuitry also affect the SAR variation in the body tissues. The influence of these heat sources are not considered in the performed simulations, since the main purpose of this chapter is to determine the effect of the IR-UWB electromagnetic field on the SAR variations.

7.2.3 Temperature Variation Based on Bio Heat Model

When exposed to an electromagnetic field, the absorbed power by the body tissues causes a temperature increase. A temperature increase exceeding 1–2 °C in the human body tissue can cause adverse health effects, such as a heat stroke [43]. In addition to the study of SAR variations, this chapter also analyses the temperature variation in the human head when it is exposed to IR-UWB transmission from an implanted transmitter. The temperature of the body tissues is modelled using the bio heat equation in (7.10) [44]:

$$Cp\frac{\delta T}{\delta t} = \nabla \cdot (k \nabla T) + \rho \cdot SAR + A - B(T - T_b) \tag{7.10}$$

where K is the thermal conductivity, Cp denotes the specific heat, A is the basal metabolic rate, B is the term associated with blood perfusion, ρ is the tissue density in $\frac{kg}{m^3}$ and $\nabla \cdot (k \nabla T)$ represents the thermal spatial diffusion term for heat transfer through conduction at temperature T in degrees Celsius. The bio heat equation in (7.10) is solved with the boundary conditions given in (7.11), namely:

$$K\frac{\delta T}{\delta n} = -h \cdot (T - T_a) \tag{7.11}$$

where T_a is the temperature of the surrounding environment, n is the unit vector normal to the surface of interest and h is the convection coefficient for heat exchange with the external environment.

The human body tries to regulate its core temperature by various mechanisms in order to keep it at approximately 37 °C. The effect of thermo regulatory mechanisms causes the tissue specific basal metabolic rate (A) and blood perfusion coefficient (B) in (7.10) to exhibit a dependency on body temperature rather than being a constant value. The basal metabolic rate is modelled using (7.12) [45]:

$$A = 1.1 \, A_0^{T-T_0} \tag{7.12}$$

where T_o is the basal temperature and A_o is the basal metabolic rate of the tissue.

The blood perfusion is only dependent on the local blood temperature. Variation of the blood perfusion with the temperature is obtained using the set of equations presented in [46]. All the heat related parameters for the calculation of temperature variation are obtained from [46].

7.3 Case Study I: Electromagnetic Effects of IR-UWB Signals for Wireless Capsule Endoscopy Applications

WCE has many advantages over the traditional wired endoscopic methods. It does not require sedation of the patient or close monitoring of the procedure by a trained hospital staff. It can potentially be used for remote monitoring of the patients from isolated locations away from hospitals. One of the most important aspects of WCE is that it is the only method of obtaining images of the small intestine, whereas the wired endoscopy devices can only reach the colon or the upper part of the digestive tract [4, 47–50]. Many reported designs for wireless endoscopy system use a narrow-band wireless link in-order to transmit image data [4, 51]. However, compared to wired endoscopy methods, existing narrowband WCE devices suffer from limited battery life, low frame rate and low resolution [52]. IR-UWB can be identified as a wireless technology that can cater the demand for high data rate, low power consumption and small form factor requirement in the WCE devices [18, 53, 54]. Because of the increased interest in IR-UWB as a potential candidate for the wireless physical layer technology in WCE applications, it is important to analyze the electromagnetic effects caused by the pulse-based transmission on the human body. Figure 7.2 depicts a WCE system that uses IR-UWB for data communication.

7.3.1 Antenna Model and WCE Device Positioning

The simulations for WCE application use the UWB antenna model used in the simulations for the head implant application. It is tuned for better performance inside the abdomen of the human anatomical model. The antenna operates at a 4 GHz center frequency with a bandwidth of approximately 1 GHz. The 4 GHz center frequency is chosen to minimize the interference from other wireless technologies, such as 5 GHz Wi-Fi in a practical scenario. The dimensions of the

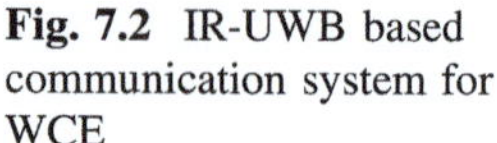

Fig. 7.2 IR-UWB based communication system for WCE

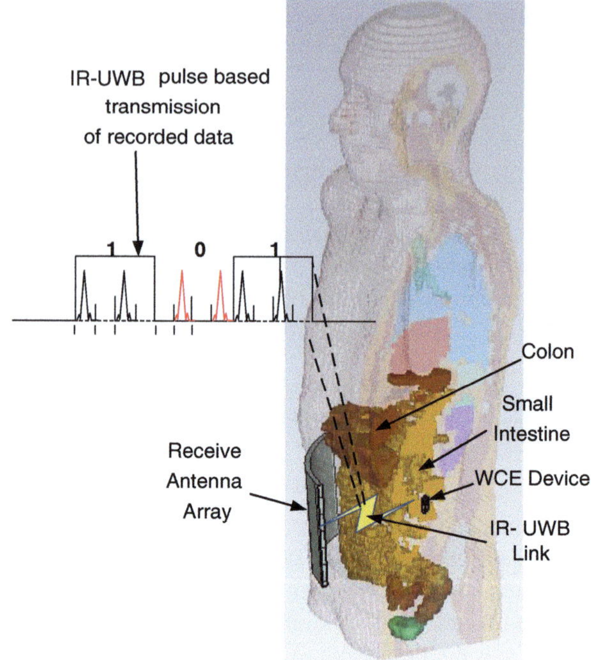

antenna model are $23.7 \times 9 \times 1.27$ mm, which are comparable with the commercially available capsule sizes used for WCE [48]. The antenna is inserted in a capsule shaped case with a diameter of 9.5 mm. The thickness of the capsule walls is negligible compared to the dimensions of the antenna. The radiating element of the antenna used in the simulations, which occupies the lower half of the antenna, is inserted in glycerin-based gel for this purpose. Glycerin has a relative permittivity of 50, which is close to the relative permittivity of the surrounding tissue material; hence allows minimal reflections of the electromagnetic wave near the transitional boundaries between the tissue medium and the capsule.

The antenna is inserted inside the small intestine, at a distance of 89 mm from the front surface of the stomach, 88 mm from the left side of the stomach, and 645 mm from the top of the head as shown in Fig. 7.3. Initially, an FCC regulated IR-UWB pulse shown in Fig. 7.4 has been used as the excitation pulse in order to investigate SAR and temperature effects. The use of an FCC regulated UWB pulse for excitation is useful to compare the obtained results with the results available in the literature. Pulses with pulse duration of 2 ns are obtained from a pulse train with a period of 50 ns. A Band Pass Filter (BPF) is used to contain the pulse power within a bandwidth of 3.5–4.5 GHz. Initially, the pulse amplitude of the signal has been adjusted ensuring that the radiated power from the antenna falls within the FCC regulated power spectrum. The power calculation is done by integrating the power spectrum of the UWB pulse in the frequency range of 3.5–4.5 GHz using

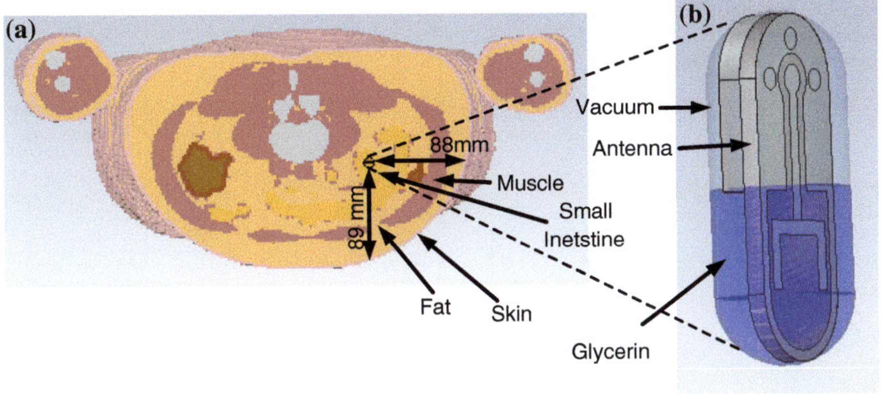

Fig. 7.3 **a** Top view simulated WCE device position **b** enlarged view of the WCE device

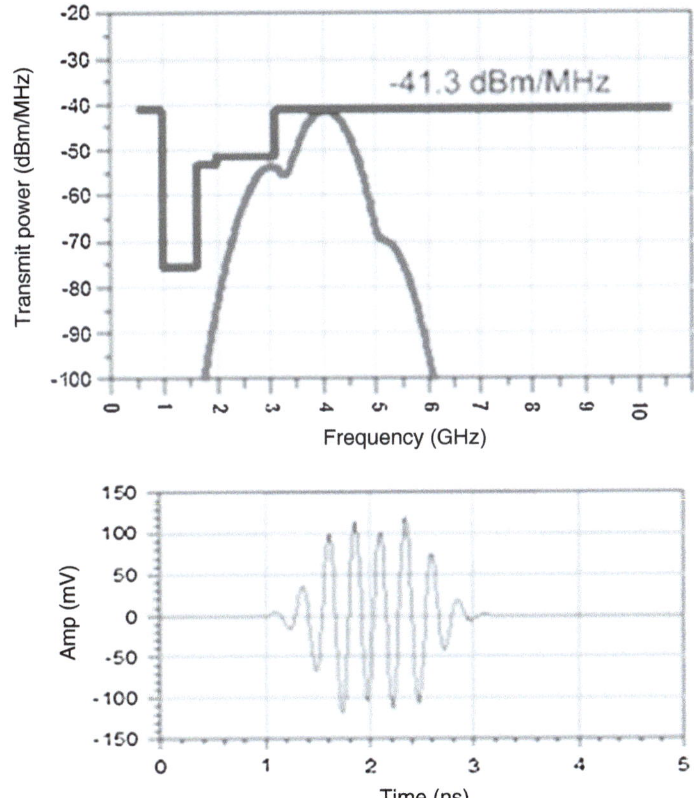

Fig. 7.4 The FCC regulated input pulse and its power spectrum

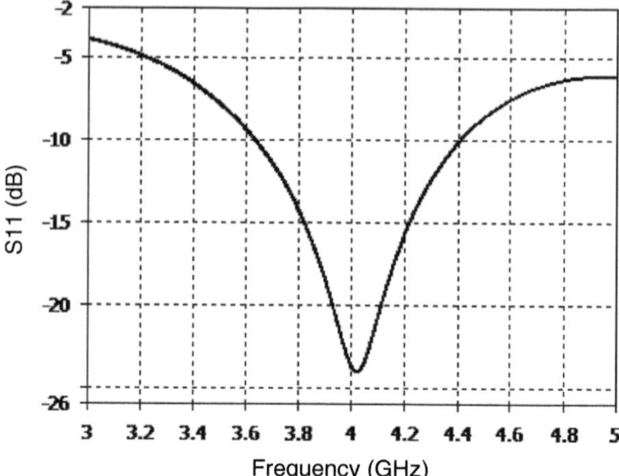

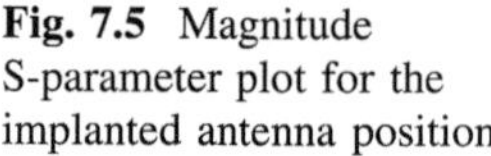

Fig. 7.5 Magnitude S-parameter plot for the implanted antenna position

the simulation software. Simulations recorded negative gain values for the antenna after tissue absorption; this means that the signal emitted in free space is lower than the radiated power from the implanted antenna. Hence, it is possible to excite the antenna with a signal power higher than the outdoor allowable 41.3 dBm/MHz power limit by increasing the excitation signal amplitude such that the power emitted to the free space after tissue absorption lies within the FCC regulations. Simulations are conducted in order to analyze the effect of this kind of manipulation on the SAR and temperature variation.

The S-parameters of the antenna for the above WCE position is depicted in Fig. 7.5. The two dimensional polar plot of the far field gain of the antenna at 4 GHz are shown in Fig. 7.6. The far field gain is shown on the x–y plane that passes through the centre of antenna. The angle (Phi) in Fig. 7.6 is measured in an anti-clockwise direction from the X-axis that passes through the centre of the antenna. The three dimensional far field antenna gain is calculated using (7.13), and converted into a two-dimensional plot using the gain values at the intersections with the x-y plane.

It can be seen from the far field results that the two-dimensional antenna gain is −63 dBi. It was observed from the simulations that the maximum three-dimensional gain is slightly higher than the two dimensional gain, and lies in the same direction. The gain is significantly low because of the large power absorption by the surrounding tissue mass. The recorded negative antenna gain after the tissue absorption means that a power level that is significantly higher than the FCC recommended spectral mask of −41.3 dBm/MHz for indoor transmission of the IR-UWB signals can be used for the antenna excitation, given that the regulations applied for SAR and SA are met [49, 50]. The delivered power to the antenna can be arranged such that the IR-UWB power level after the power loss due to tissue absorption lies within the FCC approved spectral mask. Simulations are carried out

Fig. 7.6 Antenna far field gain plot at 4 GHz (Gain (dBi) vs. Phi (degrees))

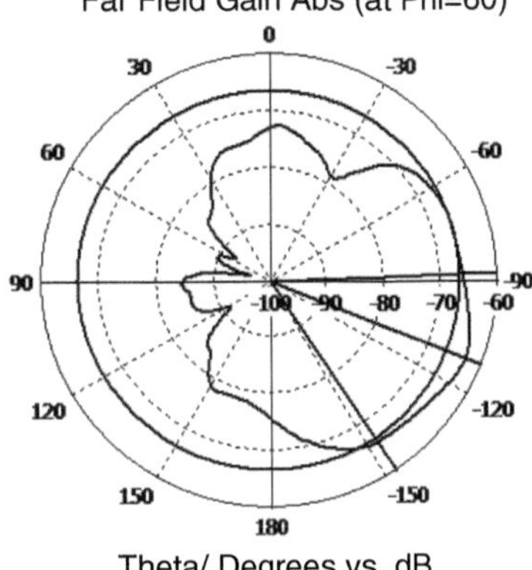

using both the FCC regulated IR-UWB pulse and an IR-UWB pulse with a power spectrum that is higher than the FCC spectral mask in order to assess and compare the SAR variations.

7.3.2 SAR, SA Variations due to the Operation of IR-UWB-Based WCE Devices

SAR and temperature simulations are carried out for different signal power levels of the WCE antenna placed at a fixed position. Figure 7.7 presents the SAR variations for the first scenario. Figure 7.7a shows the SAR variation for an IR-UWB pulse with a total in-band signal power level which lies within the FCC spectral mask of -41.3 dBm/MHz. The SAR variation in Fig. 7.7b corresponds to an IR-UWB pulse that causes a maximum 10 g averaged SAR value of 2 W/kg which is the ICNIRP allowed SAR limit. Figure 7.7c depicts the SAR variation for an IR-UWB pulse that results in a signal power level just outside the human body to lay within the FCC regulated spectral mask. The maximum SA is calculated for each scenario using (7.9). An IR-UWB pulse width of 2 ns is used for the calculation of the SA. The in-band power of the IR-UWB pulses for the three different scenarios is varied by changing the pulse amplitude. The total in-band power for each simulation is calculated by integrating the power spectrum of the IR-UWB pulse in the frequency band of 3.5–4.5 GHz. The color scale in Fig. 7.7

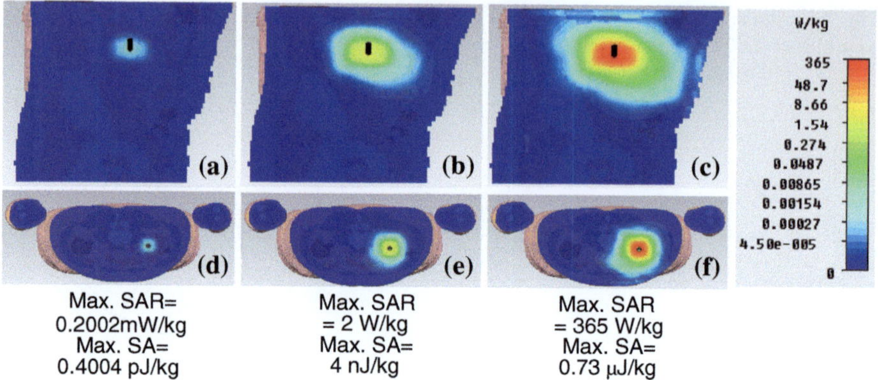

Fig. 7.7 Side view (**a–c**) and top view (**d–f**) of the simulated 10 average SAR variations in the human voxel model for IR-UWB pulses with peak spectral input power limits of (**a–d**) − 41.3 dBm/MHz (**b–e**) −1.82 dBm/MHz (**c–f**) 21.7 dBm/MHz and total in-band signal power of (**a–d**) 0.0024 mW (**b–e**) 21.5 mW (**c–f**) 4.38 W

is set to reflect the maximum SAR in all the scenarios, and is logarithmically marked to yield an acceptable resolution for low SAR values.

The results depicted in Fig. 7.7 show that the SAR variation for the third scenario, where the input signal power is adjusted in order to obtain a signal with a power level that lies within the FCC allowed spectral mask just outside the body corresponds to an SAR variation that exceeds the ICNIRP allowed level of 2 W/ kg. In other words, it can be observed from the results that it is the ICNIRP regulated SAR level of 2 W/kg that determines the maximum allowable signal power radiated from the antenna. This corresponds to an IR-UWB pulse with a total in-band signal power of 21.5 mW. The SAR variation shown in Fig. 7.7a is comparatively lower because of the small in-band power contained in the FCC regulated IR-UWB input pulse.

7.3.3 Temperature Variation Caused by IR-UWB-Based WCE Devices

The temperature variations for the same power level scenarios used for Fig. 7.7a–b are shown in Fig. 7.8. The temperature increase is obtained after the steady state is achieved. The initial body temperature is considered to be 37 °C. It can be observed from Fig. 7.8a that the temperature of the whole body has increased to 37.173 °C from the initial body temperature of 37 °C. There is no significant temperature increase in the tissues surrounding the WCE device compared to the tissues that are far away from it. This can be explained as follows: the temperature of the whole body has increased to 37.173°C due to the metabolic activities of the

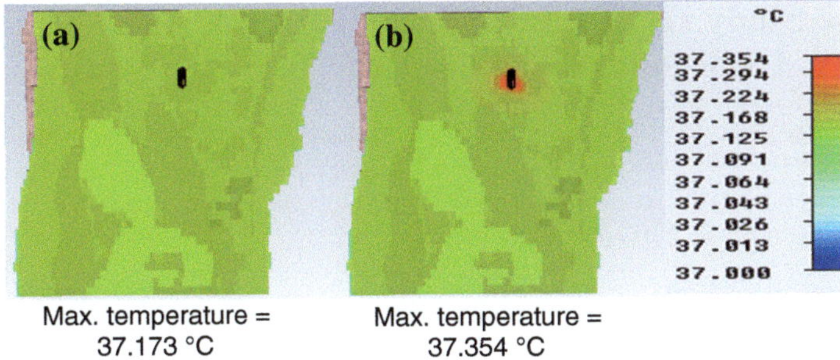

Fig. 7.8 Side view of the simulated temperature variation in the human voxel model for IR-UWB pulses with peak spectral input power limit of **a** −41.3 dBm/MHz with a total in-band signal power of 0.0024 mW **b** −1.82 dBm/MHz with a total in-band signal power 21.5 mW

Table. 7.2 SAR/SA comparison

Reference	Scenario	Body part	Reference input power	Frequency	MAX 10 g SAR/SA
[8]	In-body	Abdomen	25 mW	2.4 GHz	0.37 W/kg (SAR)
				1.2 GHz	0.64 W/kg (SAR)
				800 MHz	0.66 W/kg (SAR)
				430 MHz	0.62 W/kg (SAR)
				400 MHz	0.54 W/kg (SAR)
[22]	In-body	Abdomen	1 W (IR-UWB)	8.75 GHz	8.95 W/kg (SAR)
This study	In-body	Abdomen	−41.3 dBm/Mhz regulated IR-UWB	3.5–4.5 GHz	0.2 mW/kg (SAR) 0.4 pJ/kg (SA)
			21.5 mW (IR-UWB)		2 W/kg (SAR) 4 nJ/kg (SA)

body. The signal power of the FCC regulated delivered IR-UWB pulse is not enough to cause a significant temperature increase due to power absorption of the surrounding tissues. The blood perfusion in the human body is able to regulate the minute temperature increase caused by the small power absorption in this case. Meanwhile, the delivered pulse power for the simulations resulted in Fig. 7.8b is large enough to cause a temperature increase in the tissues at a close proximity to the WCE device. It can be observed that the temperature of the tissues at a close proximity to the WCE device has increased up to a maximum of 37.354 °C while rest of the tissues showed a temperature of 37.173 °C because of the metabolic activities. Table 7.2 compares the evaluated SAR values in this chapter with the related work in literature.

7.4 Case Study II: Electromagnetic Effects Caused by IR-UWB Signals Used in Head Implant Applications

This section presents the SAR/SA variation and temperature increase caused by IR-UWB signals used in head implant applications. This is compiled from the findings presented in [39, 51].

7.4.1 Head Implantable Antenna Model and Impedance Matching

A head implantable version of the antenna mentioned in above section is used for these simulations. The antenna is tuned to operate at around 4 GHz with a bandwidth of 1 GHz, which fulfils the bandwidth requirement imposed by the FCC for UWB communication. The antenna was inserted inside a capsule shaped casing with a negligible thickness compared to the antenna dimensions, in order to prevent direct contact between antenna radiating elements and the neighboring tissue. The radiating element of the antenna used in the simulations, which occupies the lower half of the antenna, is inserted in glycerin for the purpose of impedance matching. Glycerin has a relative permittivity of 50, which is close to the relative permittivity of the surrounding tissue material; hence allows minimal reflections of the electromagnetic wave near the transitional boundaries between the tissue medium and the capsule. The antenna is placed at 6 mm distance from the surface of the head. Figure 7.9 depicts how this antenna model is used alongside the CST voxel head model in order to perform present simulations. Through simulation-based optimization, the optimum value for the radius of the capsule ('D') was obtained to be 5 mm for the head implanted antenna, which is indicated in Fig. 7.9.

S-parameter characteristics and antenna gain/directivity far field characteristics are presented in Figs. 7.10 and 7.11, respectively. It should be noted that the near field characteristic of the antenna predominantly affects the SAR and the thermal behavior of the body tissues. The near field simulation characteristics are shown in the results section. Although the far field stretches outside of the brain and therefore does not influence the SAR, the far field characteristics are shown in order to compare the antenna performance in different scenarios as well as to get an idea about the direction in which the maximum power transfer is radiated by the antenna.

The three-dimensional far field antenna gain is calculated using the following equation:

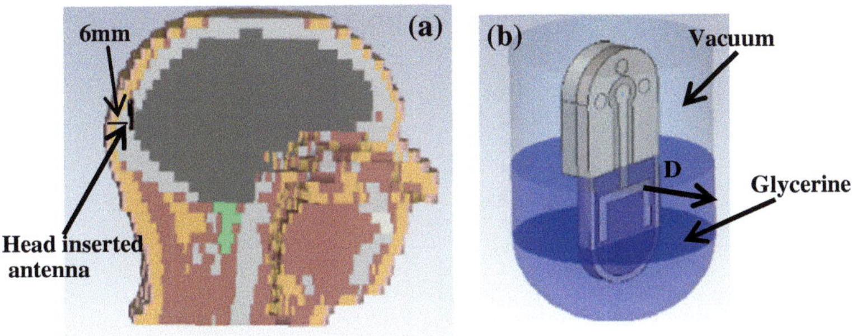

Fig. 7.9 **a** Insertion of the antenna in the head **b** IR-UWB implantable antenna

Fig. 7.10 Simulated S11 for the two different implant orientations, IEEE copyright [39]

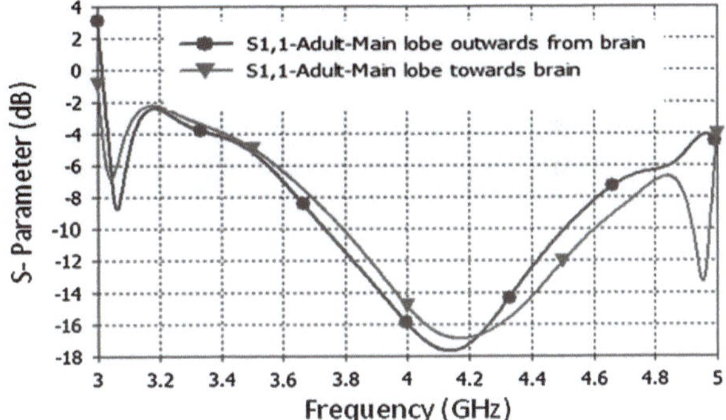

$$G = 4\pi \cdot \frac{(P_{rad} - P_{tissue})}{P_i} \qquad (7.13)$$

where G is the three dimensional gain, P_{rad} is the power radiated per unit solid angle, P_{tissue} is the power absorbed by tissues within the unit solid angle and P_i is the accepted power of the antenna after the antenna reflections. It should be noted that the antenna gain is high for antenna positions corresponding to low tissue absorptions.

7.4.2 SAR Variation for Different Signal Power Levels

10 g averaged SAR variations for three different signal power levels are analyzed for a 30-year-old adult head model using the developed simulation models (Fig. 7.11). The first scenario uses a FCC regulated IR-UWBIR-UWB pulse, which lies within the specified −41.3 dBm/MHz limit. The second scenario is obtained by considering the results in Fig. 7.11a, c: it can be observed in the latter

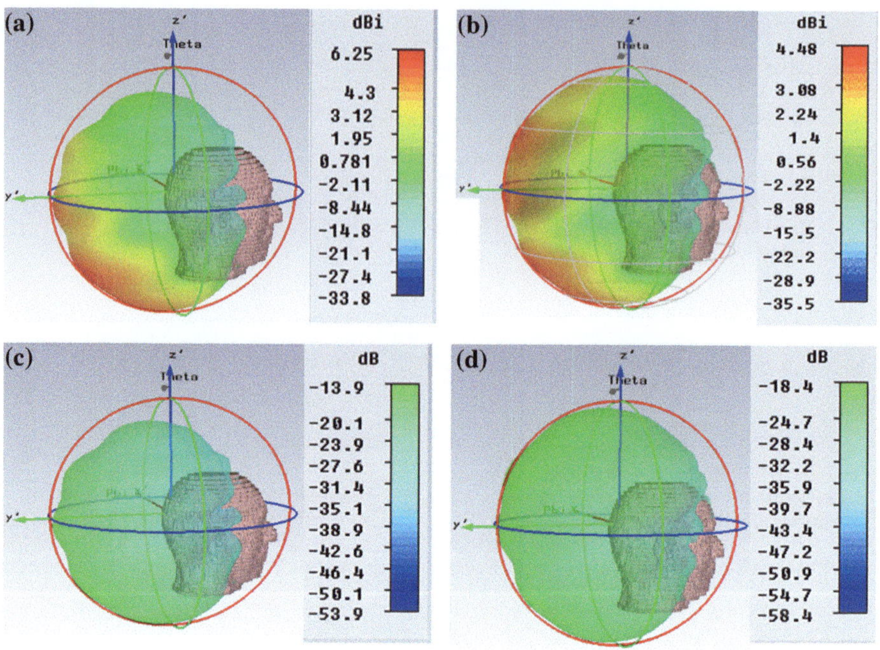

Fig. 7.11 a–b Directivity of the implanted antenna and **c–d** gain of the implanted antenna for (**a**, **c**) Antenna radiating outwards of the brain for adult head (**b, d**) Antenna radiating towards the brain for adult head

figure that the resulting maximum antennaAntenna gain is −13.9 dBi. This means that if a pulse with a peak power limit of 13.9 dB higher than the FCC regulated peak power limit of −41.3 dBm/MHz is used as the power from the implanted antenna, the radiation in free space will lie at the FCC limit. This corresponds to an input pulse with peak spectral limit of −27.4 dBm/MHz. In the third scenario, an IR-UWB pulse that causes a maximum SAR of 2 W/kg is used: the latter value is specified as the maximum allowable SAR limit by the ICNIRP regulations. The Specific Absorption (SA) in previous three scenarios is also calculated for a pulse width of 2 ns, in order to form a comparison with the ICNIRP special regulations for pulse transmissions. The results depicted in Fig. 7.12 show that the SAR and SA values obtained for the first and second scenario are well within the ICNIRP regulation limit for a single pulse of 2 W/kg and 2 mJ/kg respectively. This is due to the very small power contained in the signal (a total in-band accepted power of 0.0024 mW in scenario one and 0.0504 mW in scenario two considering a bandwidth of 1 GHz). It should be noted that the color scale is set to reflect the maximum SAR in all the scenarios, and is logarithmically marked to yield an acceptable resolution for low SAR values. The SAR variation in scenario three uses a signal which lies within a peak limit of 0.9 dBm/MHz for an amplitude

Fig. 7.12 Side view of the simulated 10 g averaged SAR variation in the adult voxel head model **a–c** when the antenna main lobe is situated outwards of the brain for the peak spectral power limits of **a** −41.3 dBm/MHz **b** −27.4 dBm/MHz and **c** 0.9 dBm/MHz **d** when the antenna main lobe is situated towards the brain for the peak spectral power limit of − 41.3 dBm/MHz

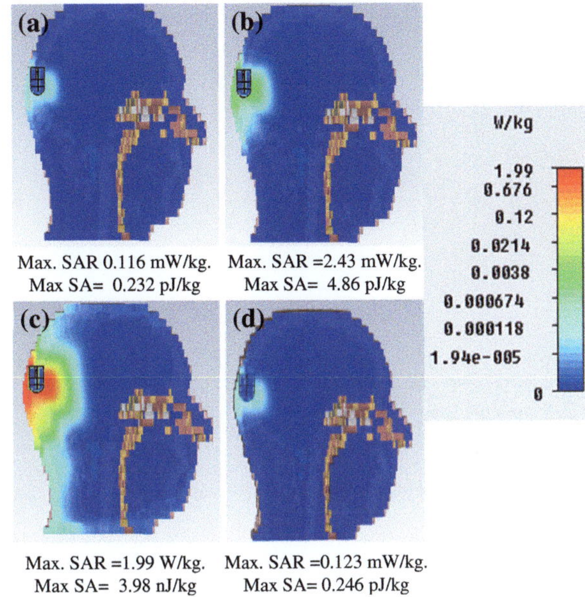

increased version of the pulse shown in Fig. 7.4, but violates the FCC regulations for IR-UWB indoor propagation.

The effect of the antenna orientation is also considered in these simulations. Two cases are considered, depending on whether the main lobe is situated outwards or inwards of the brain. In the former case, the SAR variation is obtained by placing the antenna main lobe outwards of the brain for an adult head model aged at 30 years. In the latter case, the antenna main lobe radiates towards the brain. These two scenarios are used to represent various possible applications of wireless transmission in the head. For both cases, an FCC regulated IR-UWB pulse has been considered. The results obtained are shown in Fig. 7.12a, d. The SAR value for the adult head model with the antenna main lobe pointing towards the brain is 0.007 mW/kg higher than its counterpart shown in Fig. 7.12a. This is a comparatively negligible value and is caused by the different orientations in the near field.

7.4.3 SAR Variation in Different Tissue Materials in the Human Head

The SAR variation percentages for all the tissue types involved in the simulation of the IR-UWB signal with a peak power limit of −27.4 dBm/MHz and when the antenna main lobe is located outwards from the brain are shown in Fig. 7.13: this case corresponds to the simulation depicted in Fig. 7.12c. The mass percentage of each tissue type is indicated alongside the SAR. The total SAR recorded for this

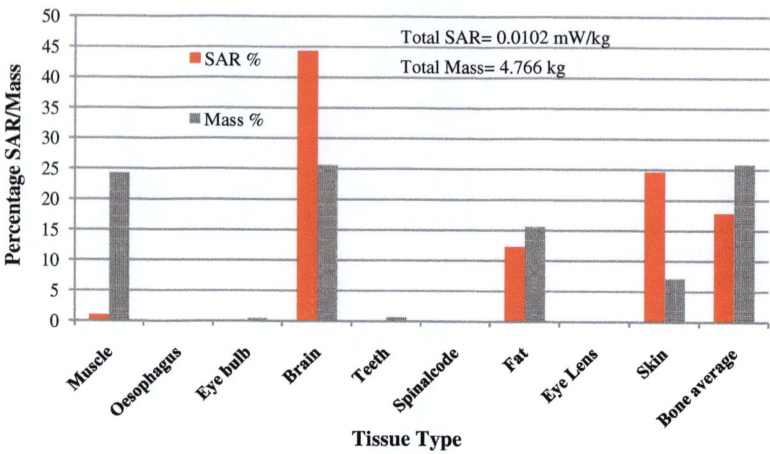

Fig. 7.13 SAR percentages and mass variation of tissue considered in the simulation, IEEE copyright [39]

scenario is 0.102 mW/kg, and the total mass of the head tissue is equal to 4.766 kg. It should be noted that the total SAR is calculated by dividing the total absorbed power by the corresponding tissue masses, unlike the calculation of the 10 g averaged SAR where local averaging over a 10 g of tissue material is considered and the maximal value is retained.

As illustrated in Fig. 7.13, brain, fat, skin and bone can be considered as tissue types with considerably high SAR percentage values. The maximum SAR percentages are recorded for the brain tissue. This is due to the fact that most of the radiated power from the antenna side lobe is directed towards the latter. The SAR percentage for the skin is relatively high considering its lower mass percentage; this is mainly due to the high water content in the former's tissue. The low water content in the bone tissue causes a comparatively low SAR value despite its comparatively high mass percentage.

7.4.4 Temperature Variation due to the Operation of IR-UWB-Based Head Implants

Simulations using the same input power scenarios as shown in Fig. 7.12a–c are used to obtain the corresponding temperature variations. The bio heat equation considers the variation of basal metabolic rate and blood perfusion. Because of the short duration of the excitation pulse, the heat conduction that occurs through sweating is assumed negligible. The temperature increase is obtained after the steady state is achieved. The initial body temperature is considered to be 37 °C. Figure 7.14 depicts the obtained temperature variations.

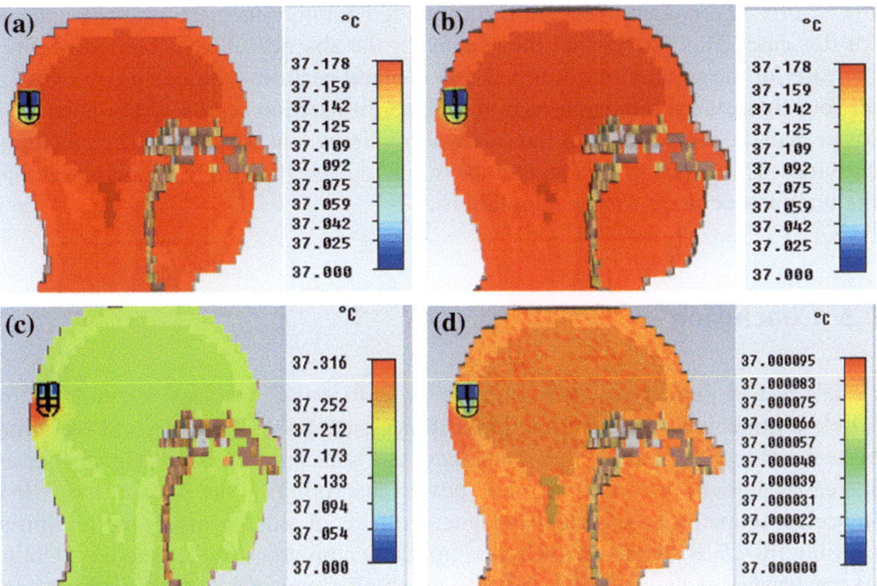

Fig. 7.14 Simulated temperature variation for a signal with peak spectral power limits of **a** −41.3 dBm/MHz **b** −27.4 dBm/MHz **c** 0.9 dBm/MHz using bio heat equation **d** −27.4 dBm/MHz without using bio heat equation, IEEE copyright [39]

It can be seen in Fig. 7.14a, b that the temperature of the whole head is increased from the initial temperature of 37–37.178 °C. It is not possible to see a significant temperature difference between the tissues at a close proximity to the antenna and those that are at a considerable distance from the antenna. This can be explained as follows. The temperature of the head as a whole increases up to 37.178 °C due to the metabolic activities in the tissues. The input powers to the antennas for cases shown in Fig. 7.14a, b are not large enough to cause a significant temperature increase due to the power absorption by the tissues. The temperature increases caused by the small radiated powers in these two cases are small enough to be regulated by the blood perfusion inside the head. This explanation is further justified by the results shown in Fig. 7.14c, d. The power delivered to the antenna for the case in Fig. 7.14c is higher than that of Fig. 7.14a, b. The high delivered power to the antenna generates a large enough electric field that causes high power absorption in the tissues. As a result, this high power absorption causes a considerable temperature increase in the tissues. It is clearly visible in Fig. 7.14c that the temperature of the tissues closer to the antenna are higher (a maximum of 37.316 °C is recorded in the simulations) than the temperature increase due to the metabolic activities in rest of the tissues (i.e. 37.178 °C). The simulations resulted in Fig. 7.14d ignore the heat generation from the metabolic activities and it does not regulate the temperature through blood perfusion. The power of the excitation pulse is set to fall within the −27.4 dBm/MHz spectral mask, which is similar to that of

Fig. 7.14b. There is an observed negligible temperature increase near the antenna for this case. This proves that the reason for the absence of a visible temperature increase for the simulations of Fig. 7.14b is blood perfusion. As can be observed in all four figures, the temperature in the glycerin insertion region of the antenna is lower than the temperature of the surrounding tissue that is heated up by metabolic activities. This is due to the fact that the initial temperature of glycerin is lower than the body temperature for the simulations.

7.5 Conclusion

IR-UWB has gained research interest as a lucrative wireless technology for wireless implant communication applications, such as WCE and neural recording systems. However, use of high frequency and wideband IR-UWB signals causes increased amount of electromagnetic power absorption by the human tissue. It is important to analyze these electromagnetic effects in order to assess the feasibility of using IR-UWB signals as a wireless implant communication technology. Unlike narrowband signals, IR-UWB signals are high frequency signals with a large bandwidth. Hence, characterizing the frequency dependent nature in the relative permittivity of the human tissue plays an important role in obtaining realistic results for electromagnetic effects caused by IR-UWB signals. This chapter describes the electromagnetic exposure effects caused by two types of UWB implanted devices used in wireless body area network applications: head implants and WCE devices. For the WCE applications of IR-UWB, it was observed that the SAR value determines the maximum IR-UWB transmit power that can be utilized in a WCE device that uses IR-UWB signals with 1 GHz bandwidth and a center frequency of 4 GHz. The maximum allowable total in-band power per pulse was found to be 21.5 mW for the particular WCE device position investigated in this chapter. The temperature increase caused by this transmit power level is discovered to be well within the control of thermal regulatory mechanisms of the human body.

For the head implant applications, the FCC regulations for the outdoor transmit power for UWB communication determines the maximum allowable signal power from an implanted IR-UWB based transmitter. It was observed for UWB based head implant applications that the SAR and SA results for the maximum peak power limit of -27.4 dBm/MHz falls within the ICNIRP regulated limits while emitting a UWB signal that falls within the FCC spectral mask when it propagates into the outdoor environment. The temperature increase due to the exposure of the head tissues to the IR-UWB electromagnetic field at those peak power limits is found to be well within the control of thermal regulatory mechanisms of the human body. Simulations also showed that it is possible to excite the antenna with a signal power higher than the outdoor allowable -41.3 dBm/MHz power limit. It was found that a pulse with a peak power limit of 13.9 dB higher than the FCC regulated peak power could be utilised for head implant applications of IR-UWB without violating SAR/SA limits, as well as the outdoor FCC regulations for this particular model.

Acknowledgment The authors would like to thank Dr. Tharaka Dissanayake for his help in designing the UWB antenna used for the high frequency simulations. Also, special thank should be given to Monash e-Research Centre, Monash University, Australia for their cooperation in assisting this work by providing the high performance computing facility for the computationally intensive simulations.

References

1. N. Gopalsami, I. Osorio, S. Kulikov, S. Buyko, A. Martynov, A.C. Raptis, SAW Microsensor Brain Implant for Prediction and Monitoring of Seizures. IEEE Sens. J. **7**(7), 977–982 (2007)
2. A.V. Nurmikko, J.P. Donoghue, L.R. Hochberg, W.R. Patterson, Y.-K. Song, C.W. Bull, D.A. Borton, F. Laiwalla, S. Park, Y. Ming, J. Aceros, Listening to brain microcircuits for interfacing with external world. Proc. IEEE Prog. Wirel. Implantable Microelectron. Neuroeng. Devices **98**(3), 375–388 (2010)
3. C. Cavallotti, M. Piccigallo, E. Susilo, P. Valdastri, A. Menciassi, P. Dario, An integrated vision system with autofocus for wireless capsular endoscopy. Sens. Actuators, A **156**(1), 72–78 (2009)
4. X. Chen, X. Zhang, L. Zhang, X. Li, N. Qi, H. Jiang, Z. Wang, A wireless capsule endoscope system with low-Power controlling and processing ASIC. IEEE Trans. Biomed. Circ. Syst. **3**(1), 11–22 (2009)
5. ICNIRP, Guidelines for Limiting to time varying electric, magnetic, and electromagnetic fields (up to 300 GHz), in *International Commission on Non-ionizing Radiation Protection*, 1997
6. Institute of Electrical and Electronics Engineers (IEEE), in *IEEE Standard for Safety Levels with Respect to Human Exposure to Radio Frequency Electromagnetic Fields, 3 kHz to 300 GHz*. IEEE Std C95.1-2005 (2005)
7. P. Soontornpipit, Effects of radiation and SAR from wireless implanted medical devices on the human body. J. Med. Assoc. Thai. **95**(2), 189–197 (2012)
8. L. Xu, M.Q.H. Meng, H. Ren, Y. Chan, Radiation characteristics of ingestible wireless devices in human intestine following radio frequency exposure at 430, 800, 1200, and 2400 MHz. IEEE Trans. Antennas Propag. **57**(8), 2418–2428 (2009)
9. Q. Wang, J. Wang, SA/SAR analysis for multiple UWB pulse exposure, in *Asia-Pacific Symposium on Electromagnetic Compatibility and 19th International Zurich Symposium on Electromagnetic Compatibility*, pp. 212–215, 19–23 May 2008
10. M. Klemm, G. Troester, EM energy absorption in the human body tissues due to UWB antennas. Prog. Electromagnet. Res. **62**, 261–280 (2006)
11. V. De Santis, M. Feliziani, F. Maradei, Safety assessment of UWB radio systems for body area network by the FD2TD method. IEEE Trans. Magn. **46**(8), 3245–3248 (2010)
12. Z.N. Chen, A. Cai, T.S.P. See, X. Qing, M.Y.W. Chia, Small planar UWB antennas in proximity of the human head. IEEE Trans. Microw. Theor. Tech. **54**(4), 1846–1857 (2006)
13. C. Buccella, V. De Santis, M. Feliziani, Prediction of temperature increase in human eyes due to RF sources. IEEE Trans. Electromagn. Compat. **49**(4), 825–833 (2007)
14. N.I.M. Yusoff, S. Khatun, S.A. AlShehri, Characterization of absorption loss for UWB body tissue propagation model, in *IEEE 9th Malaysia International Conference on Communications*, pp. 254–258, 15–17 Dec 2009

15. A. Santorelli, M. Popovic, SAR distribution in microwave breast screening: results with TWTLTLA wideband antenna, in *Seventh International Conference on Intelligent Sensors, Sensor Networks and Information Processing*, pp. 11–16, 6–9 Dec 2011
16. F. Shahrokhi, K. Abdelhalim, D. Serletis, P.L. Carlen, R. Genov, The 128-channel fully differential digital integrated neural recording and stimulation interface. IEEE Trans. Biomed. Circuits Syst. **4**(3), 149–161 (2010)
17. M. Chae, Z. Yang, M.R. Yuce, L. Hoang, W. Liu, A 128-channel 6 mW wireless neural recording IC with spike feature extraction and UWB transmitter. IEEE Trans. Neural Syst. Rehabil. Eng. **17**, 312–321 (2009)
18. Y. Gao, Y. Zheng, S. Diao, W. Toh, C. Ang, M. Je, and C. Heng, Low-power ultra-wideband wireless telemetry transceiver for medical sensor applications. IEEE Trans. Biomed. Eng. **58**(3), 768, 772 (2011)
19. K.M.S. Thotahewa, A.I. AL-Kalbani, J.-M. Redoute, M.R. Yuce, *Electromagnetic Effects of Wireless Transmission for Neural Implants, Neural Computation, Neural Devices, and Neural Prosthesis* (Springer, New York, 2014)
20. O. Novak, C. Charles, R.B. Brown, A fully integrated 19 pJ/pulse UWB transmitter for biomedical applications implemented in 65 nm CMOS technology, in *2011 IEEE International Conference on Ultra-Wideband (ICUWB)*, pp. 72–75, 14–16 Sept 2011
21. W.-N. Liu, T.-H. Lin, An energy-efficient ultra-wideband transmitter with an FIR pulse-shaping filter, in *International Symposium on VLSI Design, Automation, and Test*, pp. 1–4, 23–25 Apr 2012
22. T. Koike-Akino, SAR analysis in tissues for in vivo UWB body area networks, in *IEEE Global Telecommunications Conference*, pp. 1–6, 30 Nov–4 Dec 2009
23. P.J. Dimbylow, Fine resolution calculations of SAR in the human body for frequencies up to 3 GHz. Phys. Med. Biol. **47**(16), 2835–2846 (2002)
24. M.R. Basar, M.F.B.A. Malek, K.M. Juni, M.I.M. Saleh, M.S. Idris, L. Mohamed, N. Saudin, N.A. Mohd Affendi, A. Ali, The use of a human body model to determine the variation of path losses in the human body channel in wireless capsule endoscopy. Prog. Electromagnet. Res. **133**, 495–513 (2014)
25. D. Kurup, M. Scarpello, G. Vermeeren, W. Joseph, K. Dhaenens, F. Axisa, L. Martens, D. Vande Ginste, H. Rogier, J. Vanfleteren, In-body path loss models for implants in heterogeneous human tissues using implantable slot dipole conformal flexible antennas. EURASIP J. Wireless Commun. Netw. ISSN: 1687-1499 (2011)
26. A. Khaleghi, I. Balasingham, Improving in-body ultra wideband communication using near-field coupling of the implanted antenna. Microw. Opt. Technol. Lett. **51**(3), 585–589 (2009)
27. A. Khaleghi, R. Chávez-Santiago, I. Balasingham, Ultra-wideband statistical propagation channel model for implant sensors in the human chest. IET Microwaves Antennas Propag. **5**(15), 1805–1812 (2011)
28. CST Studio Suite™, CST AG, Germany, http://www.cst.com, 2014
29. FCC 02-48 (UWB First Report and Order), 2002
30. S. Gabriel, R.W. Lau, C. Gabriel, The dielectric properties of biological tissues: III. parametric models for the dielectric spectrum of tissues. Phys. Med. Biol. **41**(11), 2271–2293 (1996)
31. M. O'Halloran, M. Glavin, E. Jones, Frequency-dependent modelling of ultra-wideband pulses in human tissue for biomedical applications, in *IET Irish Signals and Systems Conference*, pp. 297–301 (2006)
32. S.C. DeMarco, G. Lazzi, W. Liu, J.D. Weiland, M.S. Humayun, Computed SAR and thermal elevation in a 0.25-mm 2-D model of the human eye and head in response to an implanted retinal stimulator—part I: models and methods. IEEE Trans. Antennas Propag. **51**(9), 2274–2285 (2003)
33. C. Gabriel, S. Gabriel, R.W. Lau, The dielectric properties of biological tissues: I. Literature survey. Phys. Med. Biol. **41**(11), 2231–2249 (1996)

34. A. Peyman, C. Gabriel, E.H. Grant, G. Vermeeren, L. Martens, Variation of the dielectric properties of tissues with age: the effect on the values of SAR in children when exposed to walkie–talkie devices. Phys. Med. Biol. **54**(2), 227–241 (2009)
35. C. Gabriel, Dielectric properties of biological tissue: variation with age. Bioelectromagnetics, **26**(7), 12–18 (2005)
36. J. Wang, O. Fujiwara, S. Watanabe, Approximation of aging effect on dielectric tissue properties for SAR assessment of mobile telephones. IEEE Trans. Electromagn. Compat. **48**(2), 408–413 (2006)
37. K. Lichtenecker, Die dielektrizitatskonstante naturlicher und kunstlicher mischkorper. Phys. Z. **27**, 115–158 (1926)
38. P.L. Altman, D.S. Dittmer, *Biology Data Book: Blood and Other Body Fluids* (Federation of American Societies for Experimental Biology, Washington, DC, 1974)
39. K.M.S. Thotahewa, J.M. Redoute, M.R. Yuce, SAR, SA, and temperature variation in the human head caused by IR-UWB implants operating at 4 GHz. IEEE Trans. Microw. Theory Tech. **61**, 2161–2169 (2013)
40. T. Weiland, M. Timm, I. Munteanu, A practical guide to 3-D simulation. IEEE Microwave Mag. **9**(6), 62–75 (2008)
41. M. Clement, T. Weiland, Discrete electromagnetism with finite integral technique. Prog. Electromagn. Res. **32**, 65–87 (2001)
42. IEEE C95.3-2002, Recommended practice for measurements and computations of radio frequency electromagnetic fields with respect to human exposure to such fields, 100 kHz–300 GHz, in *IEEE Standard C95.3*, 2002
43. ACGIH, Threshold limit values for chemical substances and physical agents and biological exposure indices, in *American Conference of Governmental Industrial Hygienists*, 1996
44. H.H. Pennes, Analysis of tissue and arterial blood temperatures in resting forearm. J. Appl. Physiol. **1**, 93–122 (1948)
45. M. Hoque, O.P. Gandhi, Temperature distributions in the human leg for VLF-VHF exposures at the ANSI recommended safety levels. IEEE Trans. Biomed. Eng. **35**, 442–449 (1988)
46. P. Bernardi, M. Cavagnaro, S. Pisa, E. Piuzzi, Specific absorption rate and temperature elevation in a subject exposed in the far-field of radio-frequency sources operating in the 10–900-MHz range. IEEE Trans. Biomed. Eng. **50**(3), 295–304 (2003)
47. S.H. Lee, J. Lee, Y.J. Yoon, S. Park, C. Cheon, K. Kim, S. Nam, A wideband spiral antenna for ingestible capsule endoscope systems: experimental results in a human phantom and a pig. IEEE Trans. Biomed. Eng. **58**(6), 1734–1741 (2011)
48. A. Moglia, A. Menciassi, M.O. Schurr, P. Dario, Wireless capsule endoscopy: from diagnostic devices to multipurpose robotic systems. Biomed. Microdevices **9**(2), 235–243 (2007)
49. T. Dissanayake, K.P. Esselle, M.R. Yuce, Dielectric loaded impedance matching for wideband implanted antennas. IEEE Trans. Microw. Theory Tech. **57**(10), 2480–2487 (2009)
50. K.M.S. Thotahewa, J.M. Redoute, M.R. Yuce, Electromagnetic power absorption of the human abdomen from IR-UWB based wireless capsule endoscopy devices, in *IEEE International Conference on Ultra-Wideband (ICUWB)*, pp. 79–84, 2013
51. K.M.S. Thotahewa, J.-M. Redoute, M.R. Yuce, Electromagnetic and thermal effects of IR-UWB wireless implant systems on the human head, in *35th Annual International Conference of the IEEE Engineering in Medicine and Biology Society* (*EMBC*), pp. 5179–5182, Osaka, Japan, Jul 2013
52. G. Pan, L. Wang, Swallowable wireless capsule endoscopy: Progress and technical challenges. Gastroenterol. Res. Pract. **2012** (841691), 9 (2012)
53. M.R. Yuce, T. Dissanayake, Easy-to-swallow wireless telemetry. IEEE Microw. Mag. **13**, 90–101 (2012)
54. C. Kim, S. Nooshabadi, Design of a tunable all-digital UWB pulse generator CMOS chip for wireless endoscope. IEEE Trans. on Bio-Med. Circuits Syst. **4**(2), 118–124 (2010)

Index

K. M. S. Thotahewa et al., *Ultra Wideband Wireless Body Area Networks*,
DOI: 10.1007/978-3-319-05287-8,
© Springer International Publishing Switzerland 2014